Virtual Clinical Excursions—Medical-Surgical

for

Lewis, Dirksen, Heitkemper, and Bucher
Medical-Surgical Nursing:
Assessment and Management of Clinical Problems,
Tenth Edition

Virtual Clinical Excursions—Medical-Surgical

for

Lewis, Dirksen, Heitkemper, and Bucher
Medical-Surgical Nursing:
Assessment and Management of Clinical Problems,

Tenth Edition

prepared by

Sandra J. Bleza, MSN, RN, CNE
Clinical Assistant Professor
College of Nursing and Health Professions
Valparaiso University
Valparaiso, Indiana

software developed by

Wolfsong Informatics, LLC
Tucson, Arizona

ELSEVIER

ELSEVIER

3251 Riverport Lane
Maryland Heights, Missouri 63043

VIRTUAL CLINICAL EXCURSIONS—MEDICAL-SURGICAL FOR
LEWIS, DIRKSEN, HEITKEMPER, AND BUCHER:
MEDICAL-SURGICAL NURSING: ASSESSMENT AND
MANAGEMENT OF CLINICAL PROBLEMS,
TENTH EDITION

ISBN-13: 978-0-323-37119-3

Notice

Knowledge and best practice in this field are constantly changing. As new research and experience broaden our understanding, changes in research methods, professional practices, or medical treatment may become necessary.

Practitioners and researchers must always rely on their own experience and knowledge in evaluating and using any information, methods, compounds, or experiments described herein. In using such information or methods they should be mindful of their own safety and the safety of others, including parties for whom they have a professional responsibility.

With respect to any drug or pharmaceutical products identified, readers are advised to check the most current information provided (i) on procedures featured or (ii) by the manufacturer of each product to be administered, to verify the recommended dose or formula, the method and duration of administration, and contraindications. It is the responsibility of practitioners, relying on their own experience and knowledge of their patients, to make diagnoses, to determine dosages and the best treatment for each individual patient, and to take all appropriate safety precautions.

To the fullest extent of the law, neither the Publisher nor the authors, contributors, or editors, assume any liability for any injury and/or damage to persons or property as a matter of products liability, negligence or otherwise, or from any use or operation of any methods, products, instructions, or ideas contained in the material herein.

ISBN: 978-0-323-37119-3

Printed in the United States of America

Last digit is the print number: 9 8 7 6 5 4 3 2 1

Textbook prepared by

Sharon L. Lewis, RN, PhD, FAAN
Professor Emeritus
University of New Mexico
Albuquerque, New Mexico

Former Castella Distinguished Professor
School of Nursing
University of Texas Health Science Center at San Antonio
San Antonio, Texas

Developer and Consultant
Stress-Busting Program for Family Caregivers

Shannon Ruff Dirksen, RN, PhD, FAAN
Associate Professor
College of Nursing and Health Innovation
Arizona State University
Phoenix, Arizona

Margaret McLean Heitkemper, RN, PhD, FAAN
Professor and Chairperson, Biobehavioral Nursing and Health Systems
Elizabeth Sterling Soule Endowed Chair in Nursing
School of Nursing

Adjunct Professor, Division of Gastroenterology
School of Medicine
University of Washington
Seattle, Washington

Linda Bucher, RN, PhD, CEN, CNE
Emeritus Professor
School of Nursing, University of Delaware
Newark, Delaware

Consultant/Mentor
W. Cary Edwards School of Nursing,
Thomas Edison State College
Trenton, New Jersey

Per Diem Staff Nurse
Emergency Department,
Virtua Memorial Hospital
Mt. Holly, New Jersey

Table of Contents
Virtual Clinical Excursions Workbook

Unit VIII: Problems of Ingestion, Digestion, Absorption, and Elimination

Unit IX: Problems Related to Regulatory Mechanisms

Unit X: Problems Related to Movement and Coordination

Table of Contents
Lewis, Dirksen, Heitkemper, and Bucher
Medical-Surgical Nursing:
Assessment and Management of Clinical Problems, Tenth Edition

GETTING SET UP WITH VCE ONLINE ───────────

The product you have purchased is part of the Evolve Learning System. Please read the following information thoroughly to get started.

■ HOW TO ACCESS YOUR VCE RESOURCES ON EVOLVE

There are two ways to access your VCE Resources on Evolve:

1. If your instructor has enrolled you in your VCE Evolve Resources, you will receive an email with your registration details.

2. If your instructor has asked you to self-enroll in your VCE Evolve Resources, he or she will provide you with your Course ID (for example, 1479_jdoe73_0001). You will then need to follow the instructions at https://evolve.elsevier.com/cs/studentEnroll.html.

■ HOW TO ACCESS THE ONLINE VIRTUAL HOSPITAL

The online virtual hospital is available through the Evolve VCE Resources. There is no software to download or install: the online virtual hospital runs within your Internet browser, using a pop-up window.

■ TECHNICAL REQUIREMENTS

- Broadband connection (DSL or cable)
- 1024 x 768 screen resolution
- Mozilla Firefox 18.0, Internet Explorer 9.0, Google Chrome, or Safari 5 (or higher)
  Note: Pop-up blocking software/settings must be disabled.
- Adobe Acrobat Reader
- Additional technical requirements available at http://evolvesupport.elsevier.com

■ HOW TO ACCESS THE WORKBOOK

There are two ways to access the workbook portion of *Virtual Clinical Excursions:*

1. Print workbook
2. An electronic version of the workbook, available within the VCE Evolve Resources

■ TECHNICAL SUPPORT

Technical support for *Virtual Clinical Excursions* is available by visiting the Technical Support Center at http://evolvesupport.elsevier.com or by calling 1-800-222-9570 inside the United States and Canada.

Trademarks: Windows® and Macintosh® are registered trademarks.

A QUICK TOUR

Welcome to *Virtual Clinical Excursions—Medical-Surgical*, a virtual hospital setting in which you can work with multiple complex patient simulations and also learn to access and evaluate the information resources that are essential for high-quality patient care. The virtual hospital, Pacific View Regional Hospital, has realistic architecture and access to patient rooms, a Nurses' Station, and a Medication Room.

■ BEFORE YOU START

Make sure you have your textbook nearby when you use *Virtual Clinical Excursions*. You will want to consult topic areas in your textbook frequently while working with the virtual hospital and workbook.

■ HOW TO SIGN IN

- Enter your name on the Student Nurse identification badge.
- Now choose one of the four periods of care in which to work. In Periods of Care 1 through 3, you can actively engage in patient assessment, entry of data in the electronic patient record (EPR), and medication administration. Period of Care 4 presents the day in review. Highlight and click the appropriate period of care. (For this quick tour, choose **Period of Care 1: 0730-0815**.)
- This takes you to the Patient List screen (see the *How to Select a Patient* section below). Only the patients on the Medical-Surgical Floor are available. Note that the virtual time is provided in the box at the lower left corner of the screen (0730, because we chose Period of Care 1).

Note: If you choose to work during Period of Care 4: 1900-2000, the Patient List screen is skipped because you are not able to visit patients or administer medications during the shift. Instead, you are taken directly to the Nurses' Station, where the records of all the patients on the floor are available for your review.

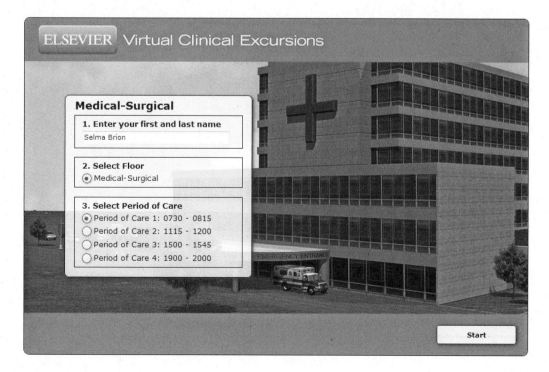

■ PATIENT LIST

MEDICAL-SURGICAL UNIT

Harry George (Room 401)
Osteomyelitis—A 54-year-old Caucasian male admitted from a homeless shelter with an infected leg. He has complications of type 2 diabetes mellitus, alcohol abuse, nicotine addiction, poor pain control, and complex psychosocial issues.

Jacquline Catanazaro (Room 402)
Asthma—A 45-year-old Caucasian female admitted with an acute asthma exacerbation and suspected pneumonia. She has complications of chronic schizophrenia, noncompliance with medication therapy, obesity, and herniated disc.

Piya Jordan (Room 403)
Bowel obstruction—A 68-year-old Asian female admitted with a colon mass and suspected adenocarcinoma. She undergoes a right hemicolectomy. This patient's complications include atrial fibrillation, hypokalemia, and symptoms of meperidine toxicity.

Clarence Hughes (Room 404)
Degenerative joint disease—A 73-year-old African-American male admitted for a left total knee replacement. His preparations for discharge are complicated by the development of a pulmonary embolus and the need for ongoing intravenous therapy.

Pablo Rodriguez (Room 405)
Metastatic lung carcinoma—A 71-year-old Hispanic male admitted with symptoms of dehydration and malnutrition. He has chronic pain secondary to multiple subcutaneous skin nodules and psychosocial concerns related to family issues with his approaching death.

Patricia Newman (Room 406)
Pneumonia—A 61-year-old Caucasian female admitted with worsening pulmonary function and an acute respiratory infection. Her chronic emphysema is complicated by heavy smoking, hypertension, and malnutrition. She needs access to community resources such as a smoking cessation program and meal assistance.

■ HOW TO SELECT A PATIENT

- You can choose one or more patients to work with from the Patient List by checking the box to the left of the patient name(s). For this quick tour, select Piya Jordan and Pablo Rodriguez. (In order to receive a scorecard for a patient, the patient must be selected before proceeding to the Nurses' Station.)
- Click on **Get Report** to the right of the medical records number (MRN) to view a summary of the patient's care during the 12-hour period before your arrival on the unit.
- After reviewing the report, click on **Go to Nurses' Station** in the right lower corner to begin your care. (*Note:* If you have been assigned to care for multiple patients, you can click on **Return to Patient List** to select and review the report for each additional patient before going to the Nurses' Station.)

Note: Even though the Patient List is initially skipped when you sign in to work for Period of Care 4, you can still access this screen if you wish to review the shift report for any of the patients. To do so, simply click on **Patient List** near the top left corner of the Nurses' Station (or click on the clipboard to the left of the Kardex). Then click on **Get Report** for the patient(s) whose care you are reviewing. This may be done during any period of care.

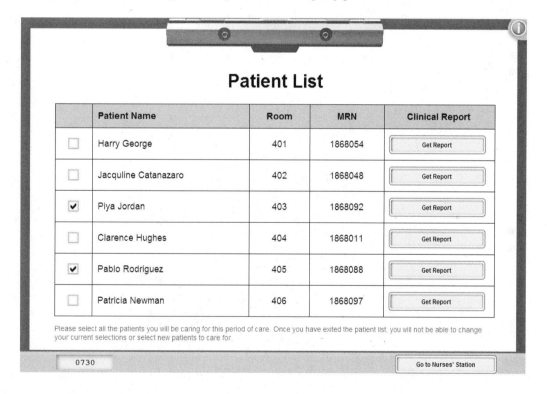

Patient List

	Patient Name	Room	MRN	Clinical Report
☐	Harry George	401	1868054	Get Report
☐	Jacquline Catanazaro	402	1868048	Get Report
☑	Piya Jordan	403	1868092	Get Report
☐	Clarence Hughes	404	1868011	Get Report
☑	Pablo Rodriguez	405	1868088	Get Report
☐	Patricia Newman	406	1868097	Get Report

Please select all the patients you will be caring for this period of care. Once you have exited the patient list, you will not be able to change your current selections or select new patients to care for.

0730   Go to Nurses' Station

■ HOW TO FIND A PATIENT'S RECORDS

NURSES' STATION

Within the Nurses' Station, you will see:

1. A clipboard that contains the patient list for that floor.
2. A chart rack with patient charts labeled by room number, a notebook labeled Kardex, and a notebook labeled MAR (Medication Administration Record).
3. A desktop computer with access to the Electronic Patient Record (EPR).
4. A tool bar across the top of the screen that can also be used to access the Patient List, EPR, Chart, MAR, and Kardex. This tool bar is also accessible from each patient's room.
5. A Drug Guide containing information about the medications you are able to administer to your patients.
6. A Laboratory Guide containing normal value ranges for all laboratory tests you may come across in the virtual patient hospital.
7. A tool bar across the bottom of the screen that can be used to access the Floor Map, patient rooms, Medication Room, and Drug Guide.

As you run your cursor over an item, it will be highlighted. To select, simply click on the item. As you use these resources, you will always be able to return to the Nurses' Station by clicking on the **Return to Nurses' Station** bar located in the right lower corner of your screen.

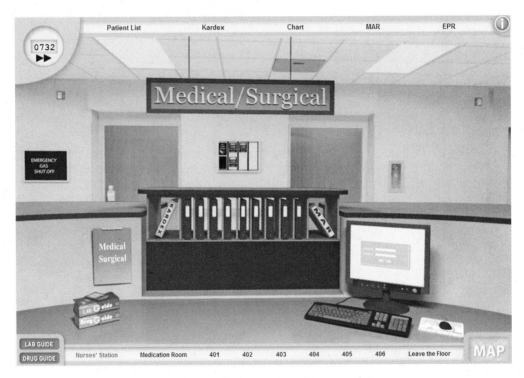

MEDICATION ADMINISTRATION RECORD (MAR)

The MAR icon located on the tool bar at the top of your screen accesses current 24-hour medications for each patient. Click on the icon and the MAR will open. (*Note:* You can also access the MAR by clicking on the MAR notebook on the far right side of the book rack in the center of the screen.) Within the MAR, tabs on the right side of the screen allow you to select patients by room number. Be careful to make sure you select the correct tab number for *your* patient rather than simply reading the first record that appears after the MAR opens. Each MAR sheet lists the following:

- Medications
- Route and dosage of each medication
- Times of administration of each medication

Note: The MAR changes each day. Expired MARs are stored in the patients' charts.

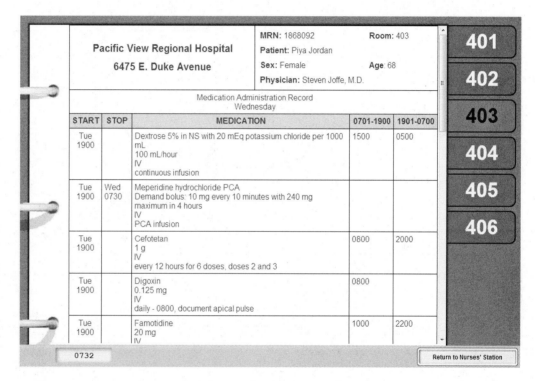

		Pacific View Regional Hospital 6475 E. Duke Avenue	MRN: 1868092 Room: 403 Patient: Piya Jordan Sex: Female Age: 68 Physician: Steven Joffe, M.D.			401 402 403 404 405 406
		Medication Administration Record Wednesday				
START	**STOP**	**MEDICATION**	**0701-1900**	**1901-0700**		
Tue 1900		Dextrose 5% in NS with 20 mEq potassium chloride per 1000 mL 100 mL/hour IV continuous infusion	1500	0500		
Tue 1900	Wed 0730	Meperidine hydrochloride PCA Demand bolus: 10 mg every 10 minutes with 240 mg maximum in 4 hours IV PCA infusion				
Tue 1900		Cefotetan 1 g IV every 12 hours for 6 doses, doses 2 and 3	0800	2000		
Tue 1900		Digoxin 0.125 mg IV daily - 0800, document apical pulse	0800			
Tue 1900		Famotidine 20 mg IV	1000	2200		

0732

Return to Nurses' Station

CHARTS

To access patient charts, either click on the **Chart** icon at the top of your screen or anywhere within the chart rack in the center of the Nurses' Station screen. When the close-up view appears, the individual charts are labeled by room number. To open a chart, click on the room number of the patient whose chart you wish to review. The patient's name and allergies will appear on the left side of the screen, along with a list of tabs on the right side of the screen, allowing you to view the following data:

- Allergies
- Physician's Orders
- Physician's Notes
- Nurse's Notes
- Laboratory Reports
- Diagnostic Reports
- Surgical Reports
- Consultations

- Patient Education
- History and Physical
- Nursing Admission
- Expired MARs
- Consents
- Mental Health
- Admissions
- Emergency Department

Information appears in real time. The entries are in reverse chronologic order, so use the down arrow at the right side of each chart page to scroll down to view previous entries. Flip from tab to tab to view multiple data fields or click on **Return to Nurses' Station** in the lower right corner of the screen to exit the chart.

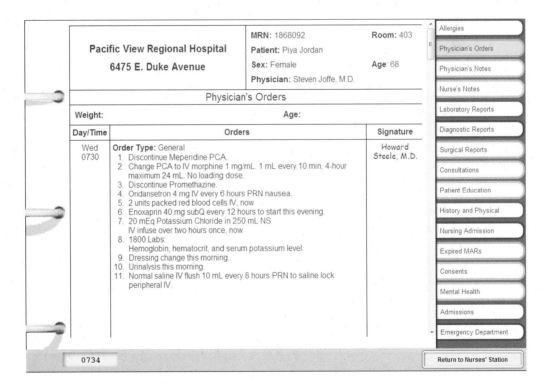

ELECTRONIC PATIENT RECORD (EPR)

The EPR can be accessed from the computer in the Nurses' Station or from the EPR icon located in the tool bar at the top of your screen. To access a patient's EPR:
- Click on either the computer screen or the **EPR** icon.
- Your username and password are automatically filled in.
- Click on **Login** to enter the EPR.
- *Note:* Like the MAR, the EPR is arranged numerically. Thus when you enter, you are initially shown the records of the patient in the lowest room number on the floor. To view the correct data for *your* patient, remember to select the correct room number, using the drop-down menu for the Patient field at the top left corner of the screen.

The EPR used in Pacific View Regional Hospital represents a composite of commercial versions being used in hospitals. You can access the EPR:
- to review existing data for a patient (by room number).
- to enter data you collect while working with a patient.

The EPR is updated daily, so no matter what day or part of a shift you are working, there will be a current EPR with the patient's data from the past days of the current hospital stay. This type of simulated EPR allows you to examine how data for different attributes have changed over time, as well as to examine data for all of a patient's attributes at a particular time. The EPR is fully functional (as it is in a real-life hospital). You can enter such data as blood pressure, breath sounds, and certain treatments. The EPR will not, however, allow you to enter data for a previous time period. Use the arrows at the bottom of the screen to move forward and backward in time.

Patient Room: 403	Category: Vital Signs			Electronic Patient Records
Name: Piya Jordan	Wed 0700	Wed 0715	Wed 0731	Code Meanings
PAIN: LOCATION	OS			
PAIN: RATING	5			
PAIN: CHARACTERISTICS	C	NN		
PAIN: VOCAL CUES	VC3			
PAIN: FACIAL CUES	FC1			
PAIN: BODILY CUES				
PAIN: SYSTEM CUES				
PAIN: FUNCTIONAL EFFECTS				
PAIN: PREDISPOSING FACTORS				
PAIN: RELIEVING FACTORS				
PCA	P			
TEMPERATURE (F)	99.6			
TEMPERATURE (C)				
MODE OF MEASUREMENT	Ty			
SYSTOLIC PRESSURE	110	149		
DIASTOLIC PRESSURE	70	94		
BP MODE OF MEASUREMENT	NIBP	NIBP		
HEART RATE	104	152		
RESPIRATORY RATE	18	32		
SpO2 (%)	95	85		
BLOOD GLUCOSE				
WEIGHT				
HEIGHT				

0731   Return to Nurses' Station

At the top of the EPR screen, you can choose patients by their room numbers. In addition, you have access to 17 different categories of patient data. To change patients or data categories, click the down arrow to the right of the room number or category.

The categories of patient data in the EPR are as follows:

- Vital Signs
- Respiratory
- Cardiovascular
- Neurologic
- Gastrointestinal
- Excretory
- Musculoskeletal
- Integumentary
- Reproductive
- Psychosocial
- Wounds and Drains
- Activity
- Hygiene and Comfort
- Safety
- Nutrition
- IV
- Intake and Output

Remember, each hospital selects its own codes. The codes used in the EPR at Pacific View Regional Hospital may be different from ones you have seen in your clinical rotations. Take some time to acquaint yourself with the codes. Within the Vital Signs category, click on any item in the left column (e.g., Pain: Characteristics). In the far-right column, you will see a list of code meanings for the possible findings and/or descriptors for that assessment area.

You will use the codes to record the data you collect as you work with patients. Click on the box in the last time column to the right of any item and wait for the code meanings applicable to that entry to appear. Select the appropriate code to describe your assessment findings and type it in the box. (*Note:* If no cursor appears within the box, click on the box again until the blue shading disappears and the blinking cursor appears.) Once the data are typed in this box, they are entered into the patient's record for this period of care only.

To leave the EPR, click on **Exit EPR** in the bottom right corner of the screen.

■ VISITING A PATIENT

From the Nurses' Station, click on the room number of the patient you wish to visit (in the tool bar at the bottom of your screen). Once you are inside the room, you will see a still photo of your patient in the top left corner. To verify that this is the correct patient, click on the **Check Armband** icon to the right of the photo. The patient's identification data will appear. If you click on **Check Allergies** (the next icon to the right), a list of the patient's allergies (if any) will replace the photo.

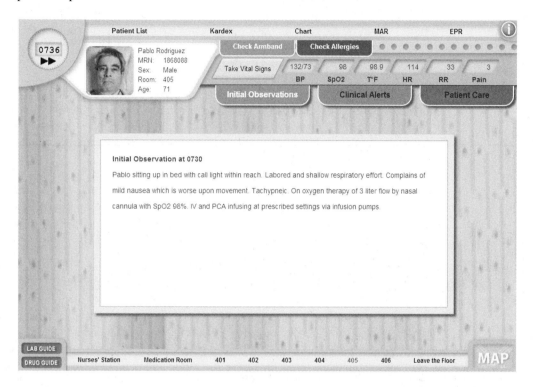

Also located in the patient's room are multiple icons you can use to assess the patient or the patient's medications. A virtual clock is provided in the upper left corner of the room to monitor your progress in real time. (*Note:* The fast-forward icon within the virtual clock will advance the time by 2-minute intervals when clicked.)

- The tool bar across the top of the screen allows you to check the **Patient List**, access the **EPR** to check or enter data, and view the patient's **Chart**, **MAR**, or **Kardex**.

- The **Take Vital Signs** icon allows you to measure the patient's up-to-the-minute blood pressure, oxygen saturation, temperature, heart rate, respiratory rate, and pain level.

- Each time you enter a patient's room, you are given an Initial Observation report to review (in the text box under the patient's photo). These notes are provided to give you a "look" at the patient as if you had just stepped into the room. You can also click on the **Initial Observations** icon to return to this box from other views within the patient's room. To the right of this icon is **Clinical Alerts**, a resource that allows you to make decisions about priority medication interventions based on emerging data collected in real time. Check this screen throughout your period of care to avoid missing critical information related to recently ordered or STAT medications.

- Clicking on **Patient Care** opens up three specific learning environments within the patient room: **Physical Assessment**, **Nurse-Client Interactions**, and **Medication Administration**.

- To perform a **Physical Assessment**, choose a body area (such as **Head & Neck**) from the column of yellow buttons. This activates a list of system subcategories for that body area (e.g., see **Sensory**, **Neurologic**, etc. in the green boxes). After you select the system you wish to evaluate, a brief description of the assessment findings will appear in a box to the right. A still photo provides a "snapshot" of how an assessment of this area might be done or what the finding might look like. For every body area, you can also click on **Equipment** on the right side of the screen.

- To the right of the Physical Assessment icon is **Nurse-Client Interactions**. Clicking on this icon will reveal the times and titles of any videos available for viewing. (*Note:* If the video you wish to see is not listed, this means you have not yet reached the correct virtual time to view that video. Check the virtual clock; you may return to access the video once its designated time has occurred—as long as you do so within the same period of care. Or you can click on the fast-forward icon within the virtual clock to advance the time by 2-minute intervals. You will then need to click again on **Patient Care** and **Nurse-Client Interactions** to refresh the screen.) To view a listed video, click on the white arrow to the right of the video title. Use the control buttons below the video to start, stop, pause, rewind, or fast-forward the action or to mute the sound.

- **Medication Administration** is the pathway that allows you to review and administer medications to a patient after you have prepared them in the Medication Room. This process is also addressed further in the *How to Prepare Medications* section below and in *Medications* in **A Detailed Tour**. For additional hands-on practice, see *Reducing Medication Errors* below **A Quick Tour** and **A Detailed Tour** in your resources.

■ HOW TO CHANGE PATIENTS OR CHANGE PERIODS OF CARE

How to Change Patients or Periods of Care: To change patients, simply click on the new patient's room number. (You cannot receive a scorecard for a new patient, however, unless you have already selected that patient on the Patient List screen.) To change to a new period of care or to restart the virtual clock, click on **Leave the Floor** and then on **Restart the Program**.

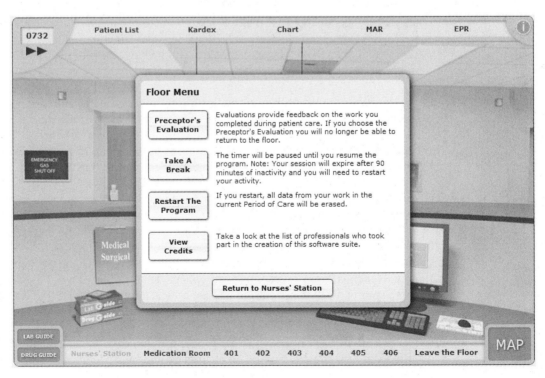

■ HOW TO PREPARE MEDICATIONS

From the Nurses' Station or the patient's room, you can access the Medication Room by clicking on the icon in the tool bar at the bottom of your screen to the left of the patient room numbers.

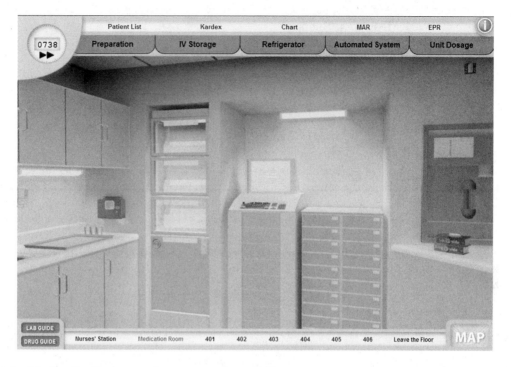

In the Medication Room you have access to the following (from left to right):

- A preparation area is located on the counter under the cabinets. To begin the medication preparation process, click on the tray on the counter or click on the **Preparation** icon at the top of the screen. The next screen leads you through a specific sequence (called the Preparation Wizard) to prepare medications one at a time for administration to a patient. However, no medication has been selected at this time. We will do this while working with a patient in **A Detailed Tour**. To exit this screen, click on **View Medication Room**.

- To the right of the cabinets (and above the refrigerator), IV storage bins are provided. Click on the bins themselves or on the **IV Storage** icon at the top of the screen. The bins are labeled **Microinfusion**, **Small Volume**, and **Large Volume**. Click on an individual bin to see a list of its contents. If you needed to prepare an IV medication at this time, you could click on the medication and its label would appear to the right under the patient's name. (*Note:* You can **Open** and **Close** any medication label by clicking the appropriate icon.) Next, you would click **Put Medication on Tray**. If you ever change your mind or decide that you have put the incorrect medication on the tray, you can reverse your actions by highlighting the medication on the tray and then clicking **Put Medication in Bin**. Click **Close Bin** in the right bottom corner to exit. **View Medication Room** brings you back to a full view of the entire room.

- A refrigerator is located under the IV storage bins to hold any medications that must be stored below room temperature. Click on the refrigerator door or on the **Refrigerator** icon at the top of the screen. Then click on the close-up view of the door to access the medications. When you are finished, click **Close Door** and then **View Medication Room**.

- To prepare controlled substances, click the **Automated System** icon at the top of the screen or click the computer monitor located to the right of the IV storage bins. A login screen will appear; your name and password are automatically filled in. Click **Login**. Select the patient for whom you wish to access medications; then select the correct medication drawer to open (they are stored alphabetically). Click **Open Drawer**, highlight the proper medication, and choose **Put Medication on Tray**. When you are finished, click **Close Drawer** and then **View Medication Room**.

- Next to the Automated System is a set of drawers identified by patient room number. To access these, click on the drawers or on the **Unit Dosage** icon at the top of the screen. This provides a close-up view of the drawers. To open a drawer, click on the room number of the patient you are working with. Next, click on the medication you would like to prepare for the patient, and a label will appear, listing the medication strength, units, and dosage per unit. To exit, click **Close Drawer**; then click **View Medication Room**.

At any time, you can learn about a medication you wish to prepare for a patient by clicking on the **Drug** icon in the bottom left corner of the medication room screen or by clicking the **Drug Guide** book on the counter to the right of the unit dosage drawers. The **Drug Guide** provides information about the medications commonly included in nursing drug handbooks. Nutritional supplements and maintenance intravenous fluid preparations are not included. Highlight a medication in the alphabetical list; relevant information about the drug will appear in the screen below. To exit, click **Return to Medication Room**.

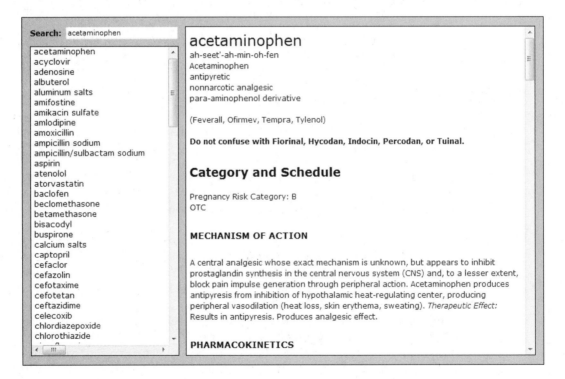

To access the MAR from the Medication Room and to review the medications ordered for a patient, click on the **MAR** icon located in the tool bar at the top of your screen and then click on the correct tab for your patient's room number. You may also click the **Review MAR** icon in the tool bar at the bottom of your screen from inside each medication storage area.

After you have chosen and prepared medications, go to the patient's room to administer them by clicking on the room number in the bottom tool bar. Inside the patient's room, click **Patient Care** and then **Medication Administration** and follow the proper administration sequence.

■ PRECEPTOR'S EVALUATIONS

When you have finished a session, click on **Leave the Floor** to go to the Floor Menu. At this point, you can click on the top icon (**Look at Your Preceptor's Evaluation**) to receive a score-card that provides feedback on the work you completed during patient care.

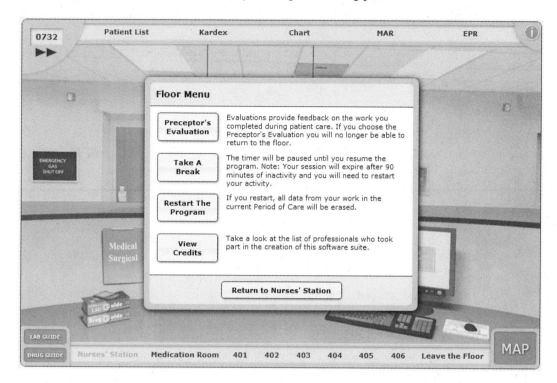

Evaluations are available for each patient you selected when you signed in for the current period of care. Click on the **Medication Scorecard** icon to see an example.

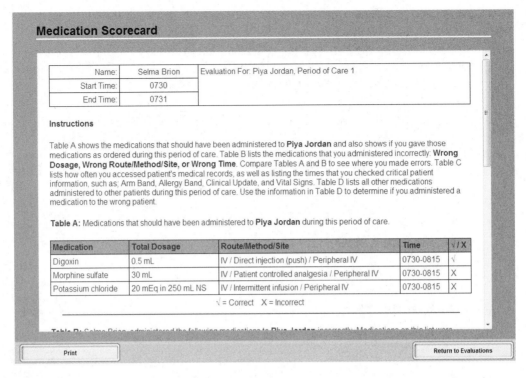

The scorecard compares the medications you administered to a patient during a period of care with what should have been administered. Table A lists the correct medications. Table B lists any medications that were administered incorrectly.

Remember, not every medication listed on the MAR should necessarily be given. For example, a patient might have an allergy to a drug that was ordered, or a medication might have been improperly transcribed to the MAR. Predetermined medication "errors" embedded within the program challenge you to exercise critical thinking skills and professional judgment when deciding to administer a medication, just as you would in a real hospital. Use all your available resources, such as the patient's chart and the MAR, to make your decision.

Table C lists the resources that were available to assist you in medication administration. It also documents whether and when you accessed these resources. For example, did you check the patient armband or perform a check of vital signs? If so, when?

You can click **Print** to get a copy of this report if needed. When you have finished reviewing the scorecard, click **Return to Evaluations** and then **Return to Menu**.

■ FLOOR MAP

To get a general sense of your location within the hospital, you can click on the **Map** icon found in the lower right corner of most of the screens in the *Virtual Clinical Excursions—Medical-Surgical* program. (*Note:* If you are following this quick tour step by step, you will need to **Restart the Program** from the Floor Menu, sign in again, and go to the Nurses' Station to access the map.) When you click the **Map** icon, a floor map appears, showing the layout of the floor you are currently on, as well as a directory of the patients and services on that floor. As you move your cursor over the directory list, the location of each room is highlighted on the map (and vice versa). The floor map can be accessed from the Nurses' Station, Medication Room, and each patient's room.

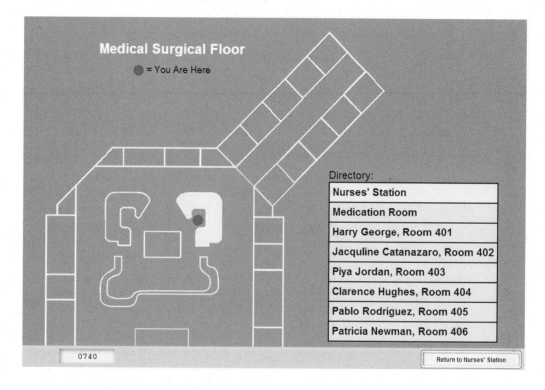

A DETAILED TOUR

If you wish to more thoroughly understand the capabilities of *Virtual Clinical Excursions—Medical-Surgical*, take a detailed tour by completing the following section. During this tour, we will work with a specific patient to introduce you to all the different components and learning opportunities available within the software.

■ WORKING WITH A PATIENT

Sign in for Period of Care 1 (0730-0815). From the Patient List, select Piya Jordan and Pablo Rodriguez; however, do not go to the Nurses' Station yet.

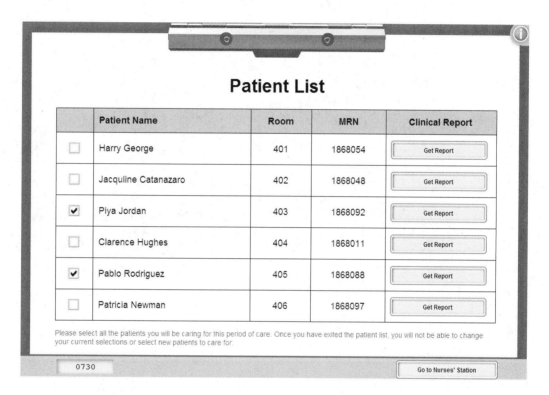

Patient List

	Patient Name	Room	MRN	Clinical Report
☐	Harry George	401	1868054	Get Report
☐	Jacquline Catanazaro	402	1868048	Get Report
☑	Piya Jordan	403	1868092	Get Report
☐	Clarence Hughes	404	1868011	Get Report
☑	Pablo Rodriguez	405	1868088	Get Report
☐	Patricia Newman	406	1868097	Get Report

Please select all the patients you will be caring for this period of care. Once you have exited the patient list, you will not be able to change your current selections or select new patients to care for.

0730   Go to Nurses' Station

■ REPORT

In hospitals, when one shift ends and another begins, the outgoing nurse who attended a patient will give a verbal and sometimes a written summary of that patient's condition to the incoming nurse who will assume care for the patient. This summary is called a report and is an important source of data to provide an overview of a patient. Your first task is to get the clinical report on Piya Jordan. To do this, click **Get Report** in the far right column in this patient's row. From a brief review of this summary, identify the problems and areas of concern that you will need to address for this patient.

When you have finished noting any areas of concern, click **Go to Nurses' Station**.

■ **CHARTS**

You can access Piya Jordan's chart from the Nurses' Station or from the patient's room (403). From the Nurses' Station, click on the chart rack or on the **Chart** icon in the tool bar at the top of your screen. Next, click on the chart labeled **403** to open the medical record for Piya Jordan. Click on the **Emergency Department** tab to view a record of why this patient was admitted.

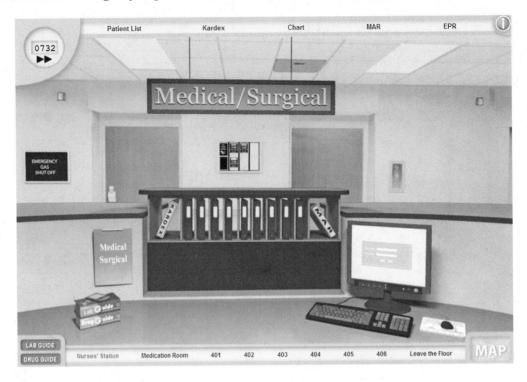

How many days has Piya Jordan been in the hospital?

What tests were done upon her arrival in the Emergency Department and why?

What was her reason for admission?

You should also click on **Diagnostic Reports** to learn what additional tests or procedures were performed and when. Finally, review the **Nursing Admission** and **History and Physical** to learn about the health history of this patient. When you are done reviewing the chart, click **Return to Nurses' Station**.

■ MEDICATIONS

Open the Medication Administration Record (MAR) by clicking on the **MAR** icon in the tool bar at the top of your screen. *Remember:* The MAR automatically opens to the first occupied room number on the floor—which is not necessarily your patient's room number! Because you need to access Piya Jordan's MAR, click on tab **403** (her room number). Always make sure you are giving the *Right Drug to the Right Patient!*

Examine the list of medications ordered for Piya Jordan. In the table below, list the medications that need to be given during this period of care (0730-0815). For each medication, note the dosage, route, and time to be given.

Time	Medication	Dosage	Route

Click on **Return to Nurses' Station**. Next, click on **403** on the bottom tool bar and then verify that you are indeed in Piya Jordan's room. Select **Clinical Alerts** (the icon to the right of Initial Observations) to check for any emerging data that might affect your medication administration priorities. Next, go to the patient's chart (click on the **Chart** icon; then click on **403**). When the chart opens, select the **Physician's Orders** tab.

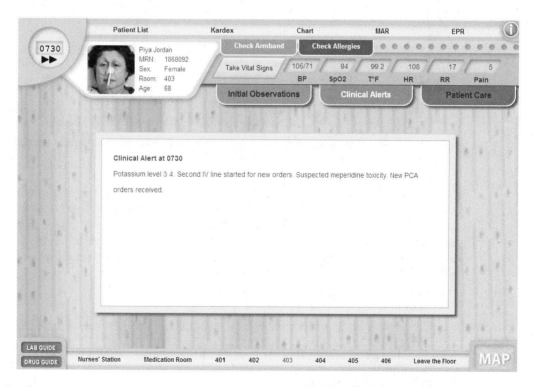

Review the orders. Have any new medications been ordered? Return to the MAR (click **Return to Room 403**; then click **MAR**). Verify that any new medications have been correctly transcribed to the MAR. Mistakes are sometimes made in the transcription process in the hospital setting, and it is sound practice to double-check any new order.

Are there any patient assessments you will need to perform before administering these medications? If so, return to Room 403 and click on **Patient Care** and then **Physical Assessment** to complete those assessments before proceeding.

Now click on the **Medication Room** icon in the tool bar at the bottom of your screen to locate and prepare the medications for Piya Jordan.

In the Medication Room, you must access the medications for Piya Jordan from the specific dispensing system in which each medication is stored. Locate each medication that needs to be given in this time period and click on **Put Medication on Tray** as appropriate. (*Hint:* Look in **Unit Dosage** drawer first.) When you are finished, click on **Close Drawer** and then on **View Medication Room**. Now click on the medication tray on the counter on the left side of the medication room screen to begin preparing the medications you have selected. (*Remember:* You can also click **Preparation** in the tool bar at the top of the screen.)

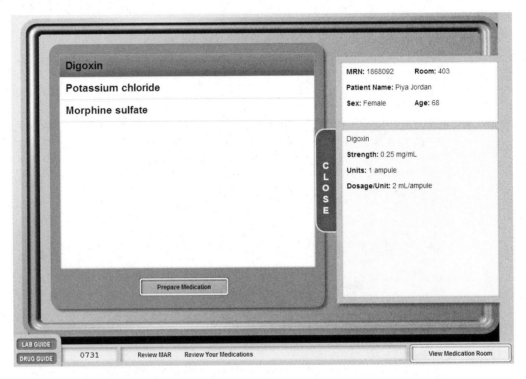

In the preparation area, you should see a list of the medications you put on the tray in the previous steps. Click on the first medication and then click **Prepare**. Follow the onscreen instructions of the Preparation Wizard, providing any data requested. As an example, let's follow the preparation process for digoxin, one of the medications due to be administered to Piya Jordan during this period of care. To begin, click to select **Digoxin**; then click **Prepare**. Now work through the Preparation Wizard sequence as detailed below:

> Amount of medication in the ampule: 2 mL.
> Enter the amount of medication you will draw up into a syringe: **0.5** mL.
> Click **Next**.
> Select the patient you wish to set aside the medication for: **Room 403, Piya Jordan**.
> Click **Finish**.
> Click **Return to Medication Room**.

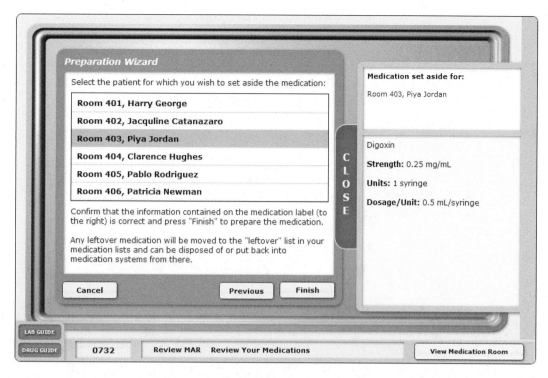

Follow this same basic process for the other medications due to be administered to Piya Jordan during this period of care. (*Hint:* Look in **IV Storage** and **Automated System**.)

Preparation Wizard Exceptions

- Some medications in *Virtual Clinical Excursions—Medical-Surgical* are preprepared by the pharmacy (e.g., IV antibiotics) and taken to the patient room as a whole. This is common practice in most hospitals.
- Blood products are not administered by students through the *Virtual Clinical Excursions—Medical-Surgical* simulations because blood administration follows specific protocols not covered in this program.
- The *Virtual Clinical Excursions—Medical-Surgical* simulations do not allow for mixing more than one type of medication, such as regular and Lente insulins, in the same syringe. In the clinical setting, when multiple types of insulin are ordered for a patient, the regular insulin is drawn up first, followed by the longer-acting insulin. Insulin is always administered in a special unit-marked syringe.

Now return to Room 403 (click on **403** on the bottom tool bar) to administer Piya Jordan's medications.

At any time during the medication administration process, you can perform a further review of systems, take vital signs, check information contained within the chart, or verify patient identity and allergies. Inside Piya Jordan's room, click **Take Vital Signs**. (*Note:* These findings change over time to reflect the temporal changes you would find in a patient similar to Piya Jordan.)

When you have gathered all the data you need, click on **Patient Care** and then select **Medication Administration**. Any medications you prepared in the previous steps should be listed on the left side of your screen. Let's continue the administration process with the digoxin ordered for Piya Jordan. Click to highlight **Digoxin** in the list of medications. Next, click on the down arrow to the right of **Select** and choose **Administer** from the drop-down menu. This will activate the Administration Wizard. Complete the Wizard sequence as follows:

- Route: **IV**
- Method: **Direct Injection**
- Site: **Peripheral IV**
- Click **Administer to Patient** arrow.
- Would you like to document this administration in the MAR? **Yes**
- Click **Finish** arrow.

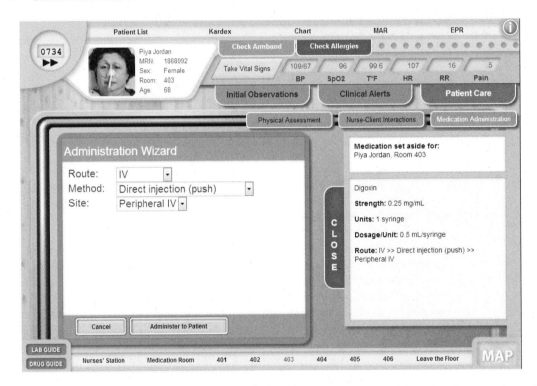

Your selections are recorded by a tracking system and evaluated on a Medication Scorecard stored under Preceptor's Evaluations. This scorecard can be viewed, printed, and given to your instructor. To access the Preceptor's Evaluations, click on **Leave the Floor**. When the Floor Menu appears, select **Look at Your Preceptor's Evaluation**. Then click on **Medication Scorecard** inside the box with Piya Jordan's name (see example on the following page).

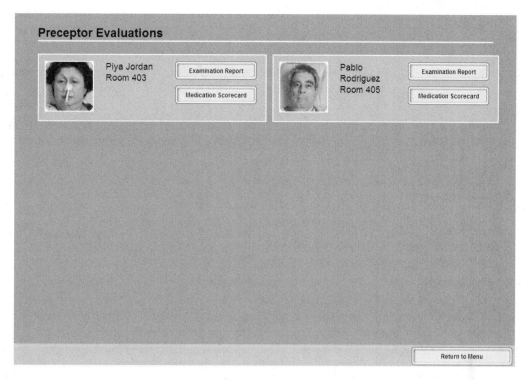

■ MEDICATION SCORECARD

- First, review Table A. Was digoxin given correctly? Did you give the other medications as ordered?
- Table B shows you which (if any) medications you gave incorrectly.
- Table C addresses the resources used for Piya Jordan. Did you access the patient's chart, MAR, EPR, or Kardex as needed to make safe medication administration decisions?
- Did you check the patient's armband to verify her identity? Did you check whether your patient had any known allergies to medications? Were vital signs taken?

When you have finished reviewing the scorecard, click **Return to Evaluations** and then **Return to Menu**.

■ VITAL SIGNS

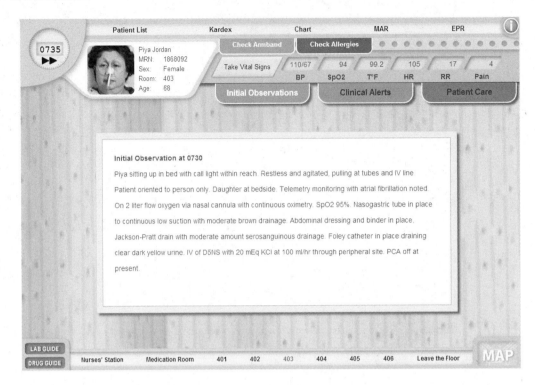

Vital signs, often considered the traditional "signs of life," include body temperature, heart rate, respiratory rate, blood pressure, oxygen saturation of the blood, and pain level.

Inside Piya Jordan's room, click **Take Vital Signs**. (*Note:* If you are following this detailed tour step by step, you will need to **Restart the Program** from the Floor Menu, sign in again for Period of Care 1, and navigate to Room 403.) Collect vital signs for this patient and record them below. Note the time at which you collected each of these data. (*Remember:* You can take vital signs at any time. The data change over time to reflect the temporal changes you would find in a patient similar to Piya Jordan.)

Vital Signs	Findings/Time
Blood pressure	
O$_2$ saturation	
Temperature	
Heart rate	
Respiratory rate	
Pain rating	

After you are done, click on the **EPR** icon located in the tool bar at the top of the screen. Your username and password are automatically provided. Click on **Login** to enter the EPR. To access Piya Jordan's records, click on the down arrow next to Patient and choose her room number, **403**. Select **Vital Signs** as the category. Next, in the empty time column on the far right, record the vital signs data you just collected in Piya Jordan's room. If you need help with this process, refer to the Electronic Patient Record (EPR) section of the Quick Tour. Now compare these findings with the data you collected earlier for this patient's vital signs. Use these earlier findings to establish a baseline for each of the vital signs.

    a.   Are any of the data you collected significantly different from the baseline for a particular vital sign?

        Circle One: Yes   No

    b.   If "Yes," which data are different?

■ PHYSICAL ASSESSMENT

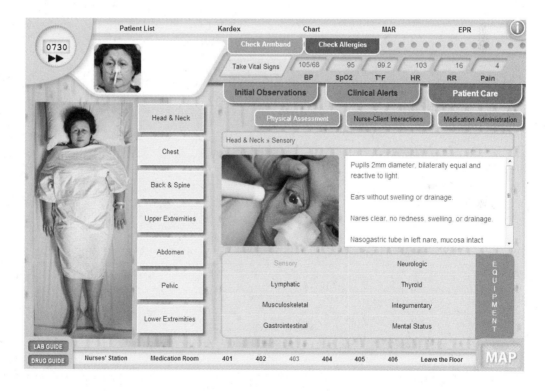

After you have finished examining the EPR for vital signs, click **Exit EPR** to return to Room 403. Click **Patient Care** and then **Physical Assessment**. Think about the information you received in the report at the beginning of this shift, as well as what you may have learned about this patient from the chart. Based on this, what area(s) of examination should you pay most attention to at this time? Is there any equipment you should be monitoring? Conduct a physical assessment of the body areas and systems that you consider priorities for Piya Jordan. For example, select **Head & Neck**; then click on and assess **Sensory** and **Lymphatic**. Complete any other assessment(s) you think are necessary at this time. In the following table, record the data you collected during this examination.

Area of Examination	Findings
Head & Neck Sensory	
Head & Neck Lymphatic	

After you have finished collecting these data, return to the EPR. Compare the data that were already in the record with those you just collected.

a. Are any of the data you collected significantly different from the baselines for this patient?

Circle One: Yes   No

b. If "Yes," which data are different?

■ NURSE-CLIENT INTERACTIONS

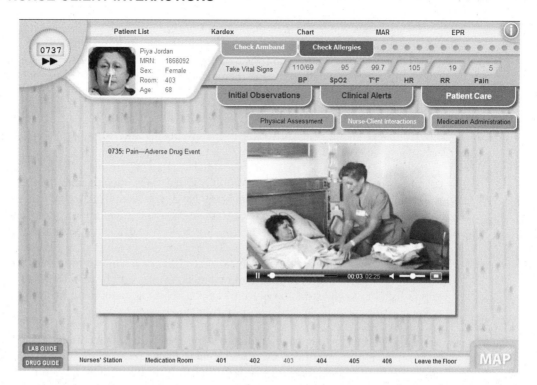

Click on **Patient Care** from inside Piya Jordan's room (403). Now click on **Nurse-Client Interactions** to access a short video titled **Pain—Adverse Drug Event**, which is available for viewing at or after 0735 (based on the virtual clock in the upper left corner of your screen; see *Note* below). To begin the video, click on the white arrow next to its title. You will observe a nurse communicating with Piya Jordan and her daughter. There are many variations of nursing practice, some exemplifying "best" practice and some not. Note whether the nurse in this interaction displays professional behavior and compassionate care. Are her words congruent with what is going on with the patient? Does this interaction "feel right" to you? If not, how would you handle this situation differently? Explain.

Note: If the video you wish to view is not listed, this means you have not yet reached the correct virtual time to view that video. Check the virtual clock; you may return to access the video once its designated time has occurred—as long as you do so within the same period of care. Or you can click on the fast-forward icon within the virtual clock to advance the time by 2-minute intervals. You will then need to click again on **Patient Care** and **Nurse-Client Interactions** to refresh the screen.

At least one Nurse-Client Interactions video is available during each period of care. Viewing these videos can help you learn more about what is occurring with a patient at a certain time and also prompt you to discern between nurse communications that are ideal and those that need improvement. Compassionate care and the ability to communicate clearly are essential components of delivering quality nursing care, and it is during your clinical time that you will begin to refine these skills.

■ **COLLECTING AND EVALUATING DATA**

Each of the activities you perform in the Patient Care environment generates a significant amount of assessment data. Remember that after you collect data, you can record your findings in the EPR. You can also review the EPR, patient's chart, videos, and MAR at any time. You will get plenty of practice collecting and then evaluating data in context of the patient's course.

Now, here's an important question for you:

> Did the previous sequence of exercises provide the most efficient way to assess Piya Jordan?

For example, you went to the patient's room to get vital signs, then back to the EPR to enter data and compare your findings with extant data. Next, you went back to the patient's room to do a physical examination, then again back to the EPR to enter and review data. If this back-and-forth process of data collection and recording seemed inefficient, remember the following:

- Plan all of your nursing activities to maximize efficiency, while at the same time optimizing the quality of patient care. (Think about what data you might need before performing certain tasks. For example, do you need to check a heart rate before administering a cardiac medication or check an IV site before starting an infusion?)

- You collect a tremendous amount of data when you work with a patient. Very few people can accurately remember all these data for more than a few minutes. Develop efficient assessment skills, and record data as soon as possible after collecting them.

- Assessment data are only the starting point for the nursing process.

Make a clear distinction between these first exercises and how you actually provide nursing care. These initial exercises were designed to involve you actively in the use of different software components. This workbook focuses on sensible practices for implementing the nursing process in ways that ensure the highest-quality care of patients.

Most important, remember that a human being changes through time, and that these changes include both the physical and psychosocial facets of a person as a living organism. Think about this for a moment. Some patients may change physically in a very short time (a patient with emerging myocardial infarction) or more slowly (a patient with a chronic illness). Patients' overall physical and psychosocial conditions may improve or deteriorate. They may have effective coping skills and familial support, or they may feel alone and full of despair. In fact, each individual is a complex mix of physical and psychosocial elements, and at least some of these elements usually change through time.

Thus it is crucial that you *DO NOT* think of the nursing process as a simple one-time, five-step procedure consisting of assessment, nursing diagnosis, planning, implementation, and evaluation. Rather, the nursing process should be utilized as a creative and systematic approach to delivering nursing care. Furthermore, because all living organisms are constantly changing, we must apply the nursing process over and over. Each time we follow the nursing process for an individual patient, we refine our understanding of that patient's physical and psychosocial conditions based on collection and analysis of many different types of data. *Virtual Clinical Excursions—Medical-Surgical* will help you develop both the creativity and the systematic approach needed to become a nurse who is equipped to deliver the highest-quality care to all patients.

REDUCING MEDICATION ERRORS ——————————————

Earlier in the detailed tour, you learned the basic steps of medication preparation and administration. The following simulations will allow you to practice those skills further—with an increased emphasis on reducing medication errors by using the Medication Scorecard to evaluate your work.

Sign in to work at Pacific View Regional Hospital for Period of Care 1. (*Note:* If you are already working with another patient or during another period of care, click on **Leave the Floor** and then **Restart the Program**; then sign in.)

From the Patient List, select Clarence Hughes. Then click on **Go to Nurses' Station**. Complete the following steps to prepare and administer medications to Clarence Hughes.

- Click on **Medication Room** on the tool bar at the bottom of your screen.
- Click on **MAR** and then on tab **404** to determine medications that have been ordered for Clarence Hughes. (*Note:* You may click on **Review MAR** at any time to verify the correct medication order. Always remember to check the patient name on the MAR to make sure you have the correct patient's record. You must click on the correct room number tab within the MAR.) Click on **Return to Medication Room** after reviewing the correct MAR.
- Click on **Unit Dosage** (or on the Unit Dosage cabinet); from the close-up view, click on drawer **404**.
- Select the medications you would like to administer. After each selection, click **Put Medication on Tray**. When you are finished selecting medications, click **Close Drawer** and then **View Medication Room**.
- Click on **Automated System** (or on the Automated System unit itself). Click **Login**.
- On the next screen, specify the correct patient and drawer location.
- Select the medication you would like to administer and click on **Put Medication on Tray**. Repeat this process if you wish to administer other medications from the Automated System.
- When you are finished, click **Close Drawer** and **View Medication Room**.
- From the Medication Room, click on **Preparation** (or on the preparation tray).
- From the list of medications on your tray, highlight the correct medication to administer and click **Prepare**.
- This activates the Preparation Wizard. Supply any requested information; then click **Next**.
- Now select the correct patient to receive this medication and click **Finish**.
- Repeat the previous three steps until all medications that you want to administer are prepared.
- You can click on **Review Your Medications** and then on **Return to Medication Room** when ready. Once you are back in the Medication Room, go directly to Clarence Hughes' room by clicking on **404** at bottom of screen.
- Inside the patient's room, administer the medication, utilizing the six rights of medication administration. After you have collected the appropriate assessment data and are ready for administration, click **Patient Care** and then **Medication Administration**. Verify that the correct patient and medication(s) appear in the left-hand window. Highlight the first medication you wish to administer; then click the down arrow next to Select. From the drop-down menu, select **Administer** and complete the Administration Wizard by providing any information requested. When the Wizard stops asking for information, click **Administer to Patient**. Specify **Yes** when asked whether this administration should be recorded in the MAR. Finally, click **Finish**.

■ **SELF-EVALUATION**

Now let's see how you did during your medication administration!

• Click on **Leave the Floor** at the bottom of your screen. From the Floor Menu, select **Look at Your Preceptor's Evaluation**. Then click **Medication Scorecard**.

The following exercises will help you identify medication errors, investigate possible reasons for these errors, and reduce or prevent medication errors in the future.

1. Start by examining Table A. These are the medications you should have given to Clarence Hughes during this period of care. If each of the medications in Table A has a ✓ by it, then you made no errors. Congratulations!

If any medication has an X by it, then you made one or more medication errors.

Compare Tables A and B to determine which of the following types of errors you made: Wrong Dose, Wrong Route/Method/Site, or Wrong Time. Follow these steps:
   a. Find medications in Table A that were given incorrectly.
   b. Now see if those same medications are in Table B, which shows what you actually administered to Clarence Hughes.
   c. Comparing Tables A and B, match the Strength, Dose, Route/Method/Site, and Time for each medication you administered incorrectly.
   d. Then, using the form below, list the medications given incorrectly and mark the errors you made for each medication.

Medication	Strength	Dosage	Route	Method	Site	Time
	❑	❑	❑	❑	❑	❑
	❑	❑	❑	❑	❑	❑
	❑	❑	❑	❑	❑	❑
	❑	❑	❑	❑	❑	❑

2. To help you reduce future medication errors, consider the following list of possible reasons for errors.

• Did not check drug against MAR for correct medication, correct dose, correct patient, correct route, correct time, correct documentation.
• Did not check drug dose against MAR three times.
• Did not open the unit dose package in the patient's room.
• Did not correctly identify the patient using two identifiers.
• Did not administer the drug on time.
• Did not verify patient allergies.
• Did not check the patient's current condition or vital sign parameters.
• Did not consider why the patient would be receiving this drug.
• Did not question why the drug was in the patient's drawer.
• Did not check the physician's order and/or check with the pharmacist when there was a question about the drug or dose.
• Did not verify that no adverse effects had occurred from a previous dose.

Based on the list of possibilities you just reviewed, determine how you made each error and record the reason in the form below:

Medication	Reason for Error

3. Look again at Table B. Are there medications listed that are not in Table A? If so, you gave a medication to Clarence Hughes that he should not have received. Complete the following exercises to help you understand how such an error might have been made.

   a. Perhaps you gave a medication that was on Clarence Hughes' MAR for this period of care, without recognizing that a change had occurred in the patient's condition, which should have caused you to reconsider. Review patient records as necessary and complete the following form:

Medication	Possible Reasons Not to Give This Medication

   b. Another possibility is that you gave Clarence Hughes a medication that should have been given at a different time. Check his MAR and complete the form below to determine whether you made a Wrong Time error:

Medication	Given to Clarence Hughes at What Time	Should Have Been Given at What Time

c. Maybe you gave another patient's medication to Clarence Hughes. In this case, you made a Wrong Patient error. Check the MARs of other patients and use the form below to determine whether you made this type of error:

Medication	Given to Clarence Hughes	Should Have Been Given to

4. The Medication Scorecard provides some other interesting sources of information. For example, if there is a medication selected for Clarence Hughes but it was not given to him, there will be an X by that medication in Table A, but it will not appear in Table B. In that case, you might have given this medication to some other patient, which is another type of Wrong Patient error. To investigate further, look at Table D, which lists the medications you gave to other patients. See whether you can find any medications ordered for Clarence Hughes that were given to another patient by mistake. However, before you make any decisions, be sure to cross-check the MAR for other patients because the same medication may have been ordered for multiple patients. Use the following form to record your findings:

Medication	Should Have Been Given to Clarence Hughes	Given by Mistake to

5. Now take some time to review the medication exercises you just completed. Use the form below to create an overall analysis of what you have learned. Once again, record each of the medication errors you made, including the type of each error. Then, for each error you made, indicate specifically what you would do differently to prevent this type of error from occurring again.

Medication	Type of Error	Error Prevention Tactic

Submit this form to your instructor if required as a graded assignment, or simply use these exercises to improve your understanding of medication errors and how to reduce them.

Name: _____   Date: _____

L E S S O N **1** _____

Culturally Competent Care

_____

Reading Assignment: Health Disparities and Culturally Competent Care (Chapter 2)

Patients: Piya Jordan, Room 403
Clarence Hughes, Room 404
Pablo Rodriguez, Room 405

Goal: To demonstrate understanding and appropriate application of cultural concepts in nursing practice.

Objectives:

1. Define *cultural competence* and associated terminology.
2. Identify appropriate methods of assessing the culture of a patient.
3. Identify specific needs for patients of various cultural and ethnic backgrounds.
4. Describe nursing interventions relevant for patients of various cultures.
5. Correctly utilize the nursing process in providing culturally competent nursing care.

In this lesson, you will explore various cultural differences and how nursing care should be adapted to meet each patient's individual needs. Begin this activity by reviewing the general concepts presented in your textbook. Answer the following questions to solidify your understanding of culture.

Exercise 1

Writing Activity

20 minutes

1. Why is it important for a nurse to assess a patient's culture?

2. Match each of the following terms with its correct definition.

Term	Definition
_____ Acculturation	a. Belief that one's own ways are superior to those of others from different cultural, ethnic, or racial backgrounds; can lead to seeing others as different or inferior.
_____ Assimilation	
_____ Cultural competence	b. A gradual process by which an individual or group learns how to take on many, but not all, values, beliefs, and practices of another culture; often results in increased similarities between the two cultures.
_____ Cultural imposition	
_____ Ethnicity	c. Viewing members of a specific culture, race, or ethnic group as being alike and sharing the same values and beliefs; can lead to false assumptions and affect a patient's care.
_____ Ethnocentrism	
_____ Stereotyping	d. Occurs when one's own cultural beliefs and practices are imposed on another person or group of people; can result in disregarding or trivializing a patient's health care beliefs or practices.

e. Refers to the manner in which an individual or group from one culture adopts certain features of another culture; typically a one-way process that may be voluntary or forced onto a group.

f. Refers to groups whose members share a common social and cultural heritage.

g. Involves the complex integration of knowledge, attitudes, and skills that enhances cross-cultural communication and fosters meaningful, respectful interactions with others.

3. Identify four processes involved in developing cultural competence.

4. Several interrelated factors influence an individual's health status. Rank the influence that the factors below have on health status from 1 to 6, with 1 being the most influential and 6 being the least influential.

_____ Genetic predisposition

_____ Environment

_____ Social circumstances

_____ Health behaviors

_____ Genetic disease

_____ Medical problems

Exercise 2

Virtual Hospital Activity

45 minutes

• Sign in to work at Pacific View Regional Hospital for Period of Care 1. (*Note:* If you are already in the virtual hospital from a previous exercise, click on **Leave the Floor** and then on **Restart the Program** to get to the sign-in window.)
• From the Patient List, select Piya Jordan (Room 403), Clarence Hughes (Room 404), and Pablo Rodriguez (Room 405).
• Click on **Go to Nurses' Station**.
• Click on **Chart** and then on **403**.
• Click on **History and Physical**.

1. Read Piya Jordan's History and Physical and document her cultural needs and/or considerations below and on the next page. Complete the table by repeating the above steps for Clarence Hughes and Pablo Rodriguez.

Patient	Cultural Needs/Considerations
Piya Jordan (Room 403)	
Clarence Hughes (Room 404)	

Patient	Cultural Needs/Considerations
Pablo Rodriguez (Room 405)	

- Click on **Return to Nurses' Station**.
- Click on **403** to enter Piya Jordan's room.
- Read the Initial Observations.
- Click on **Patient Care** and then on **Nurse-Client Interactions**.
- Select and view the video titled **0735: Pain—Adverse Drug Event**. (*Note:* Check the virtual clock to see whether enough time has elapsed. You can use the fast-forward feature to advance the time by 2-minute intervals if the video is not yet available. Then click again on **Patient Care** and **Nurse-Client Interactions** to refresh the screen.)

2. Based on this video, what potential cultural factors affecting health and health care should be identified and/or explored when planning care for Piya Jordan? (*Hint:* Use the general areas listed below to guide and organize your answer.)

Medications

Family roles and relationships

Spirituality and religion

Communication

- Click on **404** at the bottom of the screen to enter Clarence Hughes' room.
- Read the Initial Observations.
- Click on **Patient Care** and then on **Nurse-Client Interactions**.
- Select and view the video titled **0730: Assessment/Perception of Care**. (*Note:* Check the virtual clock to see whether enough time has elapsed. You can use the fast-forward feature to advance the time by 2-minute intervals if the video is not yet available. Then click again on **Patient Care** and **Nurse-Client Interactions** to refresh the screen.)

3. Based on this video, what potential cultural factors affecting health and health care should be identified and/or explored when planning care for Clarence Hughes? (*Hint:* Use the general areas listed below to guide and organize your answer.)

Religion

Communication

- Click on **405** at the bottom of the screen to enter Pablo Rodriguez's room.
- Read the Initial Observations.
- Click on **Patient Care** and then on **Nurse-Client Interactions**.
- Select and view the video titled **0730: Symptom Management**. (*Note:* Check the virtual clock to see whether enough time has elapsed. You can use the fast-forward feature to advance the time by 2-minute intervals if the video is not yet available. Then click again on **Patient Care** and **Nurse-Client Interactions** to refresh the screen.)

4. Describe how Pablo Rodriguez's comments reveal his cultural beliefs.

5. Using the nursing process, develop a culturally sensitive nursing care plan for Pablo Rodriguez in relation to the two patient problems identified in the left column below. Document your plan in the remaining columns.

Patient Problems (Assessment)	Nursing Diagnosis	Goals/Outcomes (Planning)	Nursing Interventions	Evaluation
Pain				
Spiritual/ cultural needs				

Pain

Reading Assignment: Pain (Chapter 8)

Patients: Clarence Hughes, Room 404
Pablo Rodriguez, Room 405

Goal: To demonstrate understanding and appropriate application of pain management concepts.

Objectives:

1. Define the concept of *pain*.
2. Describe the six dimensions of pain.
3. Describe the source and type of pain for each patient.
4. Perform a comprehensive pain assessment for each patient.
5. Identify variables that influence each patient's perception of pain.
6. Safely administer analgesic medications to a patient experiencing pain.
7. Plan appropriate nonpharmacologic measures that may be used to treat each patient's pain.

In this lesson, you will evaluate the pain experience of two different patients from assessment to management. Clarence Hughes is a 73-year-old male who is status post total knee arthroplasty. Pablo Rodriguez is a 71-year-old male admitted with advanced non-small cell lung carcinoma. Begin this activity by reviewing the general concepts presented in your textbook. Answer the following questions to solidify your understanding of pain.

Exercise 1

Writing Activity

10 minutes

1. Match each dimension of pain with its corresponding definition.

Pain Dimension	**Description**
_____ Affective	a. This dimension influences how painful stimuli are recognized and described. Genetic and anatomic elements are included in this dimension.
_____ Behavioral	
_____ Cognitive	b. This dimension refers to the emotional response to the pain experience.
_____ Physiologic	c. The beliefs, attitudes, memories, and meaning attributed to pain.
_____ Sociocultural	d. The observable actions used to express or control the pain experience.
	e. The demographic, support system, social roles, and cultural perspective factors associated with the pain experience.

2. Define *nociception*.

3. Place the following steps of the physiologic process in order of occurrence by numbering the steps from 1 to 4, with 1 being the first step to occur and 4 being the last.

_____ Modulation

_____ Transduction

_____ Perception

_____ Transmission

4. Which of the following statements are true in regard to the differences in pain associated with gender? Select all that apply.

_____ Women more frequently experience chronic pain such as migraine, back pain, and arthritis.

_____ Men are more likely to utilize alternative therapies to manage pain.

_____ Women are less likely to receive analgesics for chest and abdominal pain.

_____ Men report more control over pain.

_____ Men are less likely to report pain than women.

Exercise 2

Virtual Hospital Activity

45 minutes

- Sign in to work at Pacific View Regional Hospital for Period of Care 1. (*Note:* If you are already in the virtual hospital from a previous exercise, click on **Leave the Floor** and then on **Restart the Program** to get to the sign-in window.)
- From the Patient List, select Clarence Hughes (Room 404).
- Click on **Get Report**.

1. When planning care for Clarence Hughes, what roles concerning pain management may be delegated to the licensed practical/vocational nurse? Select all that apply.

_____ Develop a treatment plan for managing pain

_____ Evaluate effectiveness of prescribed pain management therapies

_____ Administer prescribed analgesics

_____ Assess pain levels

_____ Teach the patient about the prescribed pain management regimen

2. What information was obtained during report concerning Clarence Hughes' most recent pain assessment?

Now complete your own pain assessment on Clarence Hughes.

- Click on **Go to Nurses' Station**.
- Click on **404** at the bottom of the screen.
- Click on **Take Vital Signs**.

3. How does Clarence Hughes rate his pain at the present time?

- Click on **Patient Care** and then on **Physical Assessment**.
- Perform a focused assessment on Clarence Hughes by clicking on the body system categories (yellow buttons) and body system subcategories (green buttons).

4. List the findings of your focused assessment below.

- Click on **Nurse-Client Interactions**.
- Select and view the video titled **0730: Assessment/Perception of Care**. (*Note:* Check the virtual clock to see whether enough time has elapsed. You can use the fast-forward feature to advance the time by 2-minute intervals if the video is not yet available. Then click again on **Patient Care** and **Nurse-Client Interactions** to refresh the screen.)

5. How does Clarence Hughes describe his pain? Describe his nonverbal communication. Do his nonverbal cues correlate with his complaint of pain?

6. The nurse asks Clarence Hughes if she may perform an assessment before medicating him for pain. Is this appropriate? Why or why not?

- Click on **EPR** and then on **Login**.
- Select **404** from the Patient drop-down menu and select **Vital Signs** from the Category drop-down menu. (*Note:* Use the arrows at the bottom of the screen to move forward and backward in time.)
- Click on the last time column for Pain Characteristics to reveal the Code Meanings column.

7. Document Clarence Hughes' pain ratings and characteristics over the last 24 hours in the table provided below. (*Note:* The Analgesic column will be completed in question 8.)

Time of Assessment	Pain Rating	Pain Characteristic	Name of Analgesic Administered
Tuesday 0700			
Tuesday 0815			
Tuesday 0930			
Tuesday 1230			
Tuesday 1330			
Tuesday 1500			
Tuesday 1630			
Tuesday 1700			
Tuesday 2030			
Tuesday 2300			
Wednesday 0200			
Wednesday 0715			

- Click on **Exit EPR**.
- Click on **Chart** and then on **404** for Clarence Hughes' chart.
- Click on the **Expired MARs** tab.

8. Review the expired MARs for Clarence Hughes, noting the names of analgesics administered and the times of administration. Document your findings in the far right column of the table in question 7.

9. When considering the source and characteristics of Clarence Hughes' pain, what terminology can be correctly used? Select all that apply.

   _____ Superficial somatic pain

   _____ Deep somatic pain

   _____ Visceral pain

   _____ Nociceptive pain

   _____ Central pain

10. When preparing to administer oxycodone with acetaminophen, which of the following must be taken into consideration by the nurse?
    a. Hold medication if client's temperature is higher than 100° F.
    b. Hold medication if client's respiratory rate is less than 8 to 10 breaths/minute.
    c. Administer medication before meals.
    d. Administer medication with meals.

- Click on **Return to Room 404**.
- Click on **Kardex**.
- Click on **404** for Clarence Hughes' records.

11. What is the stated outcome related to comfort for Clarence Hughes? Is this a measurable outcome? How might you improve on the writing of the outcome?

12. Was the patient's pain assessed appropriately following each analgesic administration? Explain your answer. (*Hint:* Review the table you completed in question 7 of this exercise.)

13. Is the ordered analgesic medication appropriate for this type of pain? If not, what would you suggest? Are there any nonpharmacologic interventions that might be helpful for Clarence Hughes? Explain your answer.

14. What nursing assessment should be completed before administering oxycodone with acetaminophen?

15. Which of the following common side effects might Clarence Hughes experience as a result of his prescribed medication of oxycodone with acetaminophen? Select all that apply. (*Hint:* Use your textbook to answer this question rather than the Drug Guide.)

    _____ Headache

    _____ Constipation

    _____ Diarrhea

    _____ Vomiting

    _____ Sedation

    _____ Pruritus

- Click on **Return to Room 404**.
- Click on **Chart.**
- Click on **404** for Clarence Hughes' chart.
- Click on the **Nurse's Notes** tab and review the notes.

16. According to the note for Wednesday at 0715, which of the side effects that were identified in question 15 is Clarence Hughes experiencing? What should the nurse do to treat and/or prevent the analgesic-related side effect(s)?

Because Clarence Hughes received his last dose of pain medication at 0200, it is now appropriate to administer another dose. Prepare to administer a dose of analgesic to him by completing the following steps:

- Click on **Return to Room 404**.
- Click on **Medication Room** at the bottom of your screen.
- Access the **Automated System** by either selecting that icon at the top of screen or by clicking on the Automated System cart in the center of the screen.
- Click on **Login**.
- Choose Clarence Hughes in box 1 and Automated System Drawer (G-O) in box 2. Click on **Open Drawer** and review the list of available medications. (*Note:* You may click on **Review MAR** at any time to verify the medication order. Remember to look at the patient name on the MAR to make sure you have the correct record. You must click on the correct room number within the MAR. Click on **Return to Medication Room** after reviewing the correct MAR.)
- From the Open Drawer view, select the correct medication to administer. Click on **Put Medication on Tray** and then on **Close Drawer**.
- Click on **View Medication Room**.
- Begin the preparation process by clicking on **Preparation** at the top of the screen or by clicking on the tray on the counter on the left side of the Medication Room.
- Click on **Prepare**, fill in any requested data in the Preparation Wizard, and click on **Next**. Then select the correct patient and click on **Finish**.
- You can click on **Review Your Medications, on Return to Medication Room**, and then on **Prepared** when ready. Once you are back in the Medication Room, you may go directly to Clarence Hughes' room to administer this medication by clicking on **404** at the bottom of the screen.
- After you have collected the appropriate assessment data and are ready for administration, click on **Patient Care** and then on **Medication Administration**.
- Verify that the correct patient and medication(s) appear in the left-hand window.
- Click the down arrow next to Select. From the drop-down menu, select **Administer** and complete the Administration Wizard by providing any information requested.
- When the Wizard stops asking for information, click on **Administer to Patient**.
- Specify **Yes** when asked whether this administration should be recorded in the MAR.
- Finally, click on **Finish**.

Now let's see how you did!

- Click on **Leave the Floor** at the bottom of your screen.
- From the Floor Menu, select **Look at Your Preceptor's Evaluation**.
- Then click on **Medication Scorecard**.

17. Disregard the report for the routine scheduled medications but note below whether or not you correctly administered the analgesic medication. If not, why do you think you were incorrect in administering this drug? According to Table C in this scorecard, what are the appropriate resources that should be used before administering this medication? Did you utilize them correctly?

Exercise 3

Virtual Hospital Activity

45 minutes

- Sign in to work at Pacific View Regional Hospital for Period of Care 1. (*Note:* If you are already in the virtual hospital from a previous exercise, click on **Leave the Floor** and then on **Restart the Program** to get to the sign-in window.)
- From the Patient List, select Pablo Rodriguez (Room 405).
- Click on **Get Report**.

1. What was Pablo Rodriguez's pain rating at 0700, according to the change-of-shift report?

Now complete your own pain assessment on this patient.

- Click on **Go to Nurses' Station**.
- Click on **405** at the bottom of the screen.
- Click on **Take Vital Signs**.

2. How does Pablo Rodriguez rate his pain at the present time?

- Click on **Patient Care** and then on **Physical Assessment**.
- Perform a focused assessment by clicking the body system categories (yellow buttons) and body system subcategories (green buttons).

3. Document the findings from your focused assessment below.

- Click on **Chart** and then on **405**.
- Click on **Nursing Admission**. Scroll down to page 22 of the Nursing Admission form.

4. What are the aggravating and alleviating factors related to Pablo Rodriguez's pain?

- Click on **Return to Room 405**.
- Click on **Nurse-Client Interactions**.
- Select and view the video titled **0735: Patient Perceptions**. (*Note:* Check the virtual clock to see whether enough time has elapsed. You can use the fast-forward feature to advance the time by 2-minute intervals if the video is not yet available. Then click again on **Patient Care** and **Nurse-Client Interactions** to refresh the screen.)

5. What cultural influences may affect Pablo Rodriguez's perception and management of pain?

- Now scroll to review the rest of the Nursing Admission form.
- Click on **Return to Room 405**.
- Click on **Nurse-Client Interactions**.
- Select and view the video titled **0730: Symptom Management**. (*Note:* Check the virtual clock to see whether enough time has elapsed. You can use the fast-forward feature to advance the time by 2-minute intervals if the video is not yet available. Then click again on **Patient Care** and **Nurse-Client Interactions** to refresh the screen.)

- Click on **EPR** and then on **Login**.
- Select **405** from the Patient drop and **Vital Signs** from the Category drop-down menu. Use the arrows at the bottom of your screen to view vital signs previously recorded. (*Note:* You will need these data to complete question 6.)
- Click on **Exit EPR**.
- Click on **Chart** and then on **405**.
- Click on **Expired MARs** and review as needed to answer question 6.
- Click on **Return to Room 405**.
- Click on **Kardex** and then on **405** for Pablo Rodriguez's records. Review as needed to answer question 6.

6. In the table below, document Pablo Rodriguez's pain ratings, pain characteristics, the time of his medication administrations, and the orders for the analgesics administered since his admission.

Time of Assessment	Pain Rating	Pain Characteristic	Time of Medication Administration	Name of Analgesic Administered
Tues 2300				
Wed 0300				
Wed 0700				

7. What is the stated outcome related to comfort for Pablo Rodriguez? Is this a measurable outcome? How might you improve on the writing of the outcome?

8. Based on the stated outcome, the table you completed in question 6, and your pain assessment in question 2, was the pain medication administered effective? Give a rationale for your answer.

9. Was the patient's pain assessed appropriately following each analgesic administration? Explain your answer.

10. How would you classify Pablo Rodriguez's pain? Explain your answer.

11. Pablo Rodriguez's condition may reduce the effectiveness of the prescribed analgesic therapies. To increase the effectiveness of the pain management plan of treatment, adjuvant therapies may be prescribed. Discuss their use and list three agents that may be utilized.

12. _____ The nature of Pablo Rodriguez's pain places him at a high risk for addiction to the analgesics prescribed. (True/False)

13. In the 0735 video you viewed earlier in this exercise (titled **0735: Patient Perception**), the nurse asked Pablo Rodriguez about the PCA pump. Discuss the nurse's evaluation of the patient's understanding and use of the PCA pump. Do you think the nurse's actions were effective and therapeutic? If not, what other approaches would you suggest?

Palliative Care at End of Life

Reading Assignment: Palliative Care at End of Life (Chapter 9)

Patient: Pablo Rodriguez, Room 405

Goal: To demonstrate understanding and appropriate application of end-of-life concepts in nursing practice.

Objectives:

1. Identify appropriate application of palliative care concepts for a patient with a terminal illness.
2. Assess for and identify common clinical manifestations present at end of life.
3. Choose interventions appropriate to relieve clinical manifestations in a terminally ill patient.
4. Describe appropriate communication techniques when dealing with a terminally ill patient and family.
5. Discuss ethical issues related to providing pain relief during end-of-life care.

In this lesson, you will describe, plan, and evaluate the care of a patient with a terminal illness that is no longer responding to therapy. Pablo Rodriguez is a 71-year-old male suffering from advanced non-small cell lung carcinoma diagnosed 1 year ago.

Exercise 1

Writing Activity

15 minutes

1. How does the Institute of Medicine define the end of life? What are the four goals for end-of-life care?

2. What is palliative care? Describe its purpose and identify the six goals utilized during the provision of palliative care.

3. How do palliative care and hospice differ?

4. Which of the following criteria are required for admission to hospice? Select all that apply.

_____ The family must agree to participate in the delivery of care to the dying patient.

_____ The patient must desire the services.

_____ The physician must certify that the patient has 6 months or less to live.

_____ The patient must have a terminal diagnosis.

Exercise 2

Virtual Hospital Activity

45 minutes

- Sign in to work at Pacific View Regional Hospital for Period of Care 3. (*Note:* If you are already in the virtual hospital from a previous exercise, click on **Leave the Floor** and then on **Restart the Program** to get to the sign-in window.)
- From the Patient List, select Pablo Rodriguez (Room 405).
- Click on **Go to Nurses' Station**.
- Click on **Chart** and then on **405**.
- Click on the **Emergency Department** tab and review the record.

1. Why was Pablo Rodriguez admitted to the hospital?

2. What are his primary and secondary diagnoses?

• Click on **Nursing Admission**.

3. What does the admitting nurse document as this patient's anticipated needs for support at the time of discharge?

4. Does the patient have a signed advance directive?

• Click on **Nurse's Notes** and review the record.
• Click on **Return to Nurse's Station**.
• Click on **Kardex** and then on tab **405**.

5. Pablo Rodriguez is presently listed as "full code." What steps are needed to revise his status?

6. According to the textbook, what is the new term replacing a DNR (do not resuscitate) order? Describe what this term means.

- Click on **Return to Nurses' Station**.
- Click on **405** at the bottom of the screen.
- Click on **Patient Care** and then on **Nurse-Client Interactions**.
- Select and view the video titled **1530: Decision—End-of-Life Care**. (*Note:* Check the virtual clock to see whether enough time has elapsed. You can use the fast-forward feature to advance the time by 2-minute intervals if the video is not yet available. Then click again on **Patient Care** and **Nurse-Client Interactions** to refresh the screen.)

7. What is the role of the nurse when the patient and family are making decisions about code status?

8. What therapeutic communication techniques is the nurse using? Are they effective? What other technique(s) might have been used?

Exercise 3

Virtual Hospital Activity

45 minutes

- Sign in to work at Pacific View Regional Hospital for Period of Care 1. (*Note:* If you are already in the virtual hospital from a previous exercise, click on **Leave the Floor** and then on **Restart the Program** to get to the sign-in window.)
- From the Patient List, select Pablo Rodriguez (Room 405).
- Click on **Go to Nurses' Station**.
- Click on **405** at the bottom of your screen to enter Pablo Rodriguez's room.
- Read the Initial Observation.

1. According to the Initial Observation report, what physical symptom of distress is Pablo Rodriguez exhibiting?

2. How would you intervene to alleviate his symptoms? Provide rationales for your interventions.

- Click on **Nurses' Station**.
- Click on **EPR** and then on **Login**.
- Select **405** from the Patient drop-down menu and **Vital Signs** from the Category drop-down menu.

3. Describe Pablo Rodriguez's pain assessment.

4. What interventions would be appropriate to relieve this pain?

Now let's check the patient's current vital signs.

- Click on **Exit EPR**.
- Click on **405** at the bottom of your screen.
- Click on **Take Vital Signs**.

5. Based on the EPR data and Pablo Rodriguez's current pain rating, is the morphine providing effective relief? Explain.

- Click on **Patient Care** and then on **Physical Assessment**.
- Click on **Abdomen** (yellow boxes) and then on **Gastrointestinal** (green boxes).

6. Document your assessment findings below. What is the significance of these findings? How do they relate to Pablo Rodriguez's diagnosis and/or treatment?

7. How would you intervene to prevent potential complications related to the above findings?

- Click on **Nurse-Client Interactions**.
- Select and view the video titled **0730: Symptom Management**. (*Note:* Check the virtual clock to see whether enough time has elapsed. You can use the fast-forward feature to advance the time by 2-minute intervals if the video is not yet available. Then click again on **Patient Care** and **Nurse-Client Interactions** to refresh the screen.)

8. Describe Pablo Rodriguez's emotional distress as displayed in this video.

9. What nursing interventions would be appropriate to help this patient cope?

- Now select and view the video titled **0735: Patient Perceptions**. (*Note:* Check the virtual clock to see whether enough time has elapsed. You can use the fast-forward feature to advance the time by 2-minute intervals if the video is not yet available. Then click again on **Patient Care** and **Nurse-Client Interactions** to refresh the screen.)

10. Now that his pain has been controlled, what two physical symptoms does Pablo Rodriguez complain of? How would you intervene to relieve these discomforts?

11. Recall the goals for end-of-life care as noted in Exercise 1 of this lesson. Are these goals being met for Pablo Rodriguez? Explain.

Substance Abuse

Reading Assignment: Substance Abuse (Chapter 10)

Patient: Harry George, Room 401

Goal: To demonstrate understanding and appropriate application of health care concepts related to addiction and substance abuse.

Objectives:

1. Identify factors contributing to a patient's addiction.
2. Describe assessment findings related to the use of nicotine and alcohol.
3. Describe assessment findings related to withdrawal from nicotine and alcohol.
4. Examine alcohol withdrawal protocols for the care of a patient admitted to an acute care setting.
5. Identify appropriate nursing interventions when caring for a patient with substance abuse.

In this lesson, you will learn about the care of a patient undergoing specific substance abuse issues. Harry George is a 54-year-old male admitted with infection and swelling of his left foot and a history of type 2 diabetes. Begin this activity by reviewing the general concepts presented in your textbook. Answer the following questions to solidify your understanding of substance abuse.

Exercise 1

Writing Activity

10 minutes

1. Match each substance use disorder (SUD) group with its corresponding criteria.

Group	**Criteria**
_____ Impaired control	a. Presence of withdrawal symptoms when not using a substance or when using less of a substance
_____ Pharmacologic dependence	b. Missing school, work, or other responsibilities because of substance use
_____ Risky use	c. Recurrent substance use in hazardous situations
_____ Social dependence	d. Spending a great deal of time obtaining, using, or recovering from substance use

2. Which of the following substances is responsible for the greatest number of preventable illnesses and deaths each year?
   a. Caffeine
   b. Alcohol
   c. Tobacco
   d. Marijuana

3. Behaviors that may signal a substance use disorder include which of the following? Select all that apply.

   _____ Weight gain

   _____ Weight loss

   _____ Sexual dysfunction

   _____ Insomnia

   _____ Appearing older than true age

   _____ Loss of appetite

Exercise 2

Virtual Hospital Activity

30 minutes

- Sign in to work at Pacific View Regional Hospital for Period of Care 1. (*Note:* If you are already in the virtual hospital from a previous exercise, click on **Leave the Floor** and then on **Restart the Program** to get to the sign-in window.)
- From the Patient List, select Harry George (Room 401).
- Click on **Go to Nurses' Station**.
- Click on **Chart** and then on **401** to view Harry George's chart.
- Click on the **Emergency Department** tab and review this record.

1. What are Harry George's primary and secondary diagnoses?

2. What specific contributing factors to addiction are noted in the Emergency Department record? Describe how the factors contribute to alcohol abuse. (*Hint:* Read the admitting physician's notes.)

3. When did Harry George begin drinking excessively? Was there a precipitating event that contributed to this problem? If so, explain.

4. Harry George's chronic excessive use of alcohol has placed him at increased risk for alterations in health. What condition changes may result from chronic alcohol abuse? Select all that apply.

_____ Urinary retention

_____ Decreased libido

_____ Anemia

_____ Hypertension

_____ Bradycardia

5. Harry George has a history of nicotine use. Identify the 5 Rs used in the clinical assessment of a patient who is unwilling to quit using nicotine.

- Still within the chart, click on the **History and Physical** tab. Scroll to page 4 and review.

6. What assessment findings may be related to Harry George's alcohol abuse?

7. What physical examination finding may be related to cigarette smoking?

- Click on **Laboratory Reports**.

8. What is Harry George's blood alcohol level?

9. What findings can be expected based on Harry George's blood alcohol level? Select all that apply.

_____ Impaired balance

_____ Potential loss of consciousness

_____ Impaired muscle coordination

_____ Impaired judgment

_____ Significantly reduced respiration rate

- Click on **Return to Nurses' Station**.
- Click on **401** to go to Harry George's room.
- Click on **Patient Care** and then on **Nurse-Client Interactions**.
- Select and view the video titled **0735: Symptom Management**. (*Note:* Check the virtual clock to see whether enough time has elapsed. You can use the fast-forward feature to advance the time by 2-minute intervals if the video is not yet available. Then click again on **Patient Care** and **Nurse-Client Interactions** to refresh the screen.)

10. What visual assessment findings noted in this video interaction might suggest withdrawal symptoms for Harry George?

Exercise 3

Virtual Hospital Activity

45 minutes

- Sign in to work at Pacific View Regional Hospital for Period of Care 4. (*Note:* If you are already in the virtual hospital from a previous exercise, click on **Leave the Floor** and then on **Restart the Program** to get to the sign-in window.)
- Click on **Chart** and then on **401** to view Harry George's chart. (*Remember:* You are not able to visit patients or administer medications during Period of Care 4. You are able to review patients' records only.)
- Click on the **Mental Health** tab and review the record.

1. Read the Psychiatric/Mental Health Assessment for Harry George. What contributing factors to addiction are noted in this assessment?

- Click on **History and Physical**.

2. What effects of chronic alcohol abuse are present in Harry George?

3. If Harry George's alcohol abuse history were 20 years instead of just 4 years, what additional effects might occur? Identify at least one effect for each of the body systems listed below.

Central nervous system

Peripheral nervous system

Hematologic system

Musculoskeletal system

Cardiovascular system

Hepatic system

Gastrointestinal system

Urinary system

Integumentary system

- Click on **Nurse's Notes**.

4. How does the nurse describe Harry George's behavior now?

5. The textbook identifies the following symptoms of patients experiencing alcohol withdrawal. Put an X next to each symptom that applies to Harry George. Select all that apply.

_____ Tremors

_____ Anxiety

_____ Increased heart rate

_____ Increased blood pressure

_____ Nausea

_____ Sweating

_____ Hyperreflexia

_____ Insomnia

_____ Disorientation

_____ Hallucinations

_____ Increased hyperactivity without seizures

_____ Seizures

_____ Alcohol withdrawal delirium

6. Presently, Harry George's symptoms of withdrawal are categorized as minor. Listed below are the treatment options to manage the manifestations of withdrawal. Match the treatment option with the symptom it is geared to manage. (*Note:* Some treatment options may be used for multiple symptoms.)

Symptom of Withdrawal	**Treatment**
_____ Seizures	a. Benzodiazepine
_____ Tremors	b. Thiamine
_____ Wernicke's encephalopathy	c. Magnesium sulfate
_____ Visual/auditory hallucinations	d. IV glucose solution
_____ Increased blood pressure	e. Tegretol or phenytoin
_____ Increased heart rate	
_____ Hypoglycemia	
_____ Select electrolyte imbalances	

- Click on **Emergency Department**.

7. How much time has passed since Harry George had his last alcoholic drink? Calculate the number of hours that have passed since his last drink and relate this to the usual time frame noted for withdrawal symptoms.

8. Alcohol withdrawal delirium can occur within _____ to _____ days after the last drink.

- Click on **History and Physical**.

9. At the end of the History and Physical, the physician writes a plan of care. What pharmacologic interventions is the physician planning to prevent and/or treat alcohol withdrawal?

10. What is the intended benefit of thiamine administration for this patient?

11. What is the classification of chlordiazepoxide? Identify this drug's most common brand name. What is the intended therapeutic effect of this drug for Harry George? (*Hint:* For help, consult the Drug Guide located in the Nurses' Station.)

• Still in the chart, click on **Nurse's Notes**.

12. Read the notes dated Wednesday at 1245 and at 1315. Is the chlordiazepoxide effective? Give a rationale for your answer.

13. What is the classification of lorazepam? Identify its most common brand name. What is the intended therapeutic effect of this drug for Harry George?

14. Are there any potential drug interactions between chlordiazepoxide and lorazepam? If so, please describe.

15. Because both chlordiazepoxide and lorazepam are ordered for a similar therapeutic effect, what factors would influence the nurse's decision regarding which of these medications to use. (*Hint:* Consult the MAR.)

• Click on **Physician's Orders**.

16. What is the most recent physician order?

• Click on **Physician's Notes**.

17. Read the most recent physician's progress note. What is the rationale for writing the order you identified in question 16?

• Once again, click on **Nurse's Notes**.

18. Read the note for Wednesday at 1800. What clinical manifestations of nicotine withdrawal is the patient exhibiting?

19. The symptoms of nicotine withdrawal will typically occur in _____ to _____ hours.

20. How long has Harry George been without cigarettes? (*Hint:* Look at time and date of first nurse's note.)

21. What is the effect of simultaneous alcohol and nicotine withdrawal?

22. What manifestations are commonly found with nicotine withdrawal? Select all that apply.

_____   Hypertension

_____   Bradycardia

_____   Headache

_____   Restlessness

_____   Insomnia

_____   Fatigue

23. To plan nursing care for Harry George, identify three priority nursing diagnoses for the patient problems identified in the table below. For each diagnosis, identify related patient outcomes and appropriate nursing interventions to achieve these outcomes.

Patient Problems (Assessment)	Nursing Diagnosis	Goals/Outcomes (Planning)	Nursing Interventions
Tremors			
Anxiety			
Malnutrition			

LESSON 5

Cancer

Reading Assignment: Cancer (Chapter 15)
Lower Respiratory Problems (Chapter 27)
Hematologic Problems (Chapter 30)

Patient: Pablo Rodriguez, Room 405

Goal: To utilize the nursing process to competently care for patients with cancer.

Objectives:

1. Describe clinical manifestations and treatment for a patient with cancer.
2. Recognize special needs of patients undergoing treatment for cancer.
3. Appropriately treat a patient's symptoms related to disease process and/or side effects of treatment.
4. Discuss medications prescribed for a patient, including both expected therapeutic effects and adverse/side effects.
5. Plan appropriate general interventions to prevent and/or treat complications related to chemotherapy.

In this lesson, you will learn the essentials of caring for a patient diagnosed with cancer. You will collect data and assess, plan, implement, and evaluate care given. Pablo Rodriguez is a 71-year-old male admitted with advanced non-small cell lung carcinoma. Begin this lesson by reviewing the general concepts of cancer as presented in your textbook.

Exercise 1

Writing Activity

20 minutes

1. Below, match each term with its corresponding definition.

Term	Definition
_____ Carcinogen	a. The time after chemotherapy, during which the bone marrow activity and peripheral blood cell counts are at their lowest levels. Occurs at 7 to 10 days for most chemotherapy drugs.
_____ Initiation	
_____ Nadir	b. A mutation in the cell's genetic structure resulting from an error that occurs during DNA replication (inherited mutation) or following exposure to a chemical, radiation, or viral agent.
_____ Oncogene	
_____ Progression	c. The final stage in the natural history of cancer, characterized by increased growth rate of the tumor and increased invasiveness and metastasis.
_____ Promotion	
	d. Characterized by the reversible proliferation of mutated cells.
	e. A cancer-causing agent capable of producing cellular alterations that can be chemical, radiation, viral, or genetic in nature.
	f. A tumor-inducing gene.

2. Briefly define and describe the latent period.

3. What are the four types of therapies used to treat cancer? Describe the mechanism of action for each therapy.

4. What are some common side effects associated with radiation and chemotherapy?

5. Which of the following statements are correct in regard to gender differences related to cancer? Select all that apply.

_____ Thyroid cancer is more common in women than in men.

_____ The mortality rate for lung cancer is higher in women than in men.

_____ More men than women die from cancer-related deaths each year.

_____ Women are more likely to have colon cancer screenings than are men.

_____ Head and neck cancer occurs more frequently in men than in women.

Exercise 2

Virtual Hospital Activity

35 minutes

- Sign in to work at Pacific View Regional Hospital for Period of Care 1. (*Note:* If you are already in the virtual hospital from a previous exercise, click on **Leave the Floor** and then on **Restart the Program** to get to the sign-in window.)
- From the Patient List, select Pablo Rodriguez (Room 405).
- Click on **Go to Nurses' Station**.
- Click on **Chart** and then on **405**.
- Click on **History and Physical**.

1. What is Pablo Rodriguez's primary diagnosis?

2. How long ago was he diagnosed?

3. What risk factor for lung cancer is documented in the History and Physical?

4. Which are considered risk factors for the development of lung cancer? Select all that apply.

   _____ Hispanic heritage

   _____ Use of unfiltered cigarettes

   _____ Exposure to coal dust

   _____ Exposure to radon

   _____ Exposure to secondhand smoke

5. What clinical manifestations documented in the physician's review of systems are related to this disease process?

6. What treatment has Pablo Rodriguez received so far?

7. How long ago did he receive his last chemotherapy treatment?

8. What is the mechanism of action of docetaxel?

9. Patients receiving systemic chemotherapy are at an increased risk for bone marrow suppression. For each condition listed below, what specific assessments should the nurse monitor?

Neutropenia

Thrombocytopenia

Anemia

10. What interventions would be appropriate to prevent complications of bone marrow suppression?

Neutropenia

Thrombocytopenia

Anemia

• Click on **Emergency Department** in the chart.

11. Scroll down to the Emergency Department physician's progress notes for Tuesday 1800. What type of cancer was noted on the bronchoscopy performed 1 year ago? Is this a small cell cancer or non-small cell cancer?

Exercise 3

Virtual Hospital Activity

30 minutes

- Sign in to work at Pacific View Regional Hospital for Period of Care 1. (*Note:* If you are already in the virtual hospital from a previous exercise, click on **Leave the Floor** and then on **Restart the Program** to get to the sign-in window.)
- From the Patient List, select Pablo Rodriguez (Room 405).
- Click on **Get Report** and read the change-of-shift report.

1. What unresolved problem is noted in the report?

- Click on **Go to Nurses' Station**.
- Click on **Chart** and then on **405**.
- Click on **Nurse's Notes**.

2. Look at the note for Wednesday at 0415. How did the nurse respond to Pablo Rodriguez's complaints? Were the nurse's actions appropriate?

- Click on **Return to Nurses' Station**.
- Go to the patient's room by clicking on **405** at the bottom of the screen.
- Click on **Patient Care** and then on **Nurse-Client Interactions**.
- Select and view the video titled **0730: Symptom Management**. (*Note:* Check the virtual clock to see whether enough time has elapsed. You can use the fast-forward feature to advance the time by 2-minute intervals if the video is not yet available. Then click again on **Patient Care** and **Nurse-Client Interactions** to refresh the screen.)

3. What are Pablo Rodriguez's two major concerns at this point?

4. What other assessment should you do before treating the patient's complaint of nausea?

- Click on **MAR**; then click on **405** to access Pablo Rodriguez's record.

5. What medications are ordered to manage the patient's nausea?

6. What might the nurse question regarding these medication orders?

- Click on **Return to Room 405**.
- Click on **Chart** and then on **405**.
- Click on **Nursing Admission**.

7. What is the patient's weight? What is this in kilograms?

- Click on **Return to Room 405**.
- Click on the **Drug** icon in the lower left corner of the screen.

8. Calculate the maximum 24-hour dose for patients receiving this drug for nausea related to chemotherapy.

9. Calculate the maximum 24-hour dose of this drug for management of postoperative nausea and vomiting.

10. Calculate the maximum amount of this medication that Pablo Rodriguez could receive in 24 hours as ordered. Is it within the dosage guidelines? Is there any reason to be concerned about this dosage schedule over long periods of time?

11. What are the possible ramifications of giving high doses of this drug?

12. What are the ramifications of *not* giving this medication for this patient's nausea?

13. If the nurse administers the prn medication for nausea/vomiting at 0730, what should be done with the regularly scheduled 0800 dose?

Exercise 4

Virtual Hospital Activity

40 minutes

- Sign in to work at Pacific View Regional Hospital for Period of Care 2. (*Note:* If you are already in the virtual hospital from a previous exercise, click on **Leave the Floor** and then on **Restart the Program** to get to the sign-in window.)
- From the Patient List, select Pablo Rodriguez (Room 405).
- Click on **Go to Nurses' Station**.
- Click on **Chart** and then on **405**.
- Click on **Laboratory Reports**.

1. Below, record Pablo Rodriguez's alkaline phosphatase and calcium levels obtained on Tuesday at 2000.

- Click on **Return to Nurses' Station**.
- Click on **Lab Guide** on the desk.

2. Use the Lab Guide to evaluate whether the results are normal or abnormal.

3. What medications still need to be given to this patient during the day shift (up to today at 1500)?

- Click on **Return to Nurses' Station**.
- Click on the **Drug Guide** in the lower left corner of the screen.
- Use the Drug Guide to answer the next three questions.

4. How does ondansetron differ from metoclopramide in regard to antiemetic mechanism of action?

5. The rate of infusion for the IV ondansetron would be:
   a. 5 minutes.
   b. 10 minutes.
   c. 15 minutes.
   d. 20 minutes.

6. What is the expected benefit that Pablo Rodriguez will receive from dexamethasone? Over what time period should it be administered?

- Click on **Return to Nurses' Station**.
- Click on **Chart** and then on **405**.
- Click on **Patient Education**.

7. Has any teaching yet been completed? In your opinion, what teaching is a priority and should have been completed on admission?

- Click on **Return to Nurses' Station**.
- Go to Pablo Rodriguez's room by clicking on **405** at the bottom of your screen.
- Click on **Patient Care** and then on **Nurse-Client Interactions**.
- Select and view the video titled **1150: Assessment—Pain**. (*Note:* Check the virtual clock to see whether enough time has elapsed. You can use the fast-forward feature to advance the time by 2-minute intervals if the video is not yet available. Then click again on **Patient Care** and **Nurse-Client Interactions** to refresh the screen.)

8. Why is the patient not eating?

9. Is this a normal side effect of chemotherapy?

10. How would you treat this?

- Click on **Kardex** and then on **405** and read the outcomes.

11. What additional outcome(s) might you include for this patient?

12. What is the patient's code status? How do you feel about this in relation to the patient's diagnosis and condition? What is the nurse's professional responsibility related to the patient's code status?

Fluid Imbalance

Reading Assignment: Fluid, Electrolyte, and Acid-Base Imbalances (Chapter 16)

Patients: Piya Jordan, Room 403
Patricia Newman, Room 406

Goal: To utilize the nursing process to competently care for patients with fluid imbalances.

Objectives:

1. Identify normal physiologic influences on fluid and electrolyte balance.
2. Compare and contrast causes and clinical manifestations related to extracellular fluid (ECF) volume deficit and extracellular fluid excess.
3. Utilize laboratory data and clinical manifestations to assess fluid balance and imbalance.
4. Describe collaborative management strategies used to maintain and/or restore fluid balance.
5. Critically analyze differences in the fluid balance assessment findings of two patients.
6. Develop an appropriate plan of care for patients displaying extracellular fluid volume imbalances.

In this lesson, you will assess, plan, and implement care for two patients with similar but differing extracellular fluid volume imbalances. Piya Jordan is a 68-year-old female admitted with nausea and vomiting for several days following weeks of poor appetite and increasing weakness. Patricia Newman is a 61-year-old female admitted with dyspnea at rest, cough, and fever. Begin this activity by reviewing the general concepts of fluid homeostasis as presented in your textbook. Answer the following questions to cement your understanding of the normal physiologic concepts related to fluid balance.

Exercise 1

Writing Activity

20 minutes

1. Identify the two major fluid compartments in the body and describe their composition.

2. Match each cause or manifestation with the type of fluid volume condition with which it is associated.

Cause or Manifestation	**Type of Fluid Volume Condition**
_____ Confusion	a. Extracellular fluid volume deficit
_____ Diarrhea	b. Extracellular fluid volume excess
_____ Hemorrhage	c. Both extracellular fluid volume deficit and excess
_____ Seizure	
_____ Congestive heart failure	
_____ Delayed capillary refill	
_____ Peripheral edema	
_____ Long-term use of corticosteroids	

3. Match each of the following terms related to fluid volume regulation with its corresponding definition.

Term	Definition
_____ Hydrostatic pressure	a. Movement of molecules from an area of high concentration to one of low concentration
_____ Oncotic pressure	
_____ Diffusion	b. Movement of water between two compartments separated by a membrane permeable to water but not to solutes; water moves from an area of low solute concentration (dilute) to one of high solute concentration (concentrated)
_____ Osmolarity	
_____ Aldosterone	c. The force of pressure exerted by static water in a confined space—"water-pushing" pressure
_____ Hypotonic	
_____ Osmosis	d. The total milliosmoles of solute per unit of total volume of solution (mOsm/L); pertains to fluids outside the body
_____ Antidiuretic hormone	e. The solid particle dissolved in a solution
_____ Isotonic	f. Any solution with a solute concentration equal to the osmolarity of normal body fluids or normal saline, about 300 mOsm/L
_____ Solute	
_____ Facilitated diffusion	g. A hormone produced by the hypothalamus and released by the posterior pituitary gland to regulate body water
_____ Hypertonic	
_____ Active transport	h. Molecules combine with a specific carrier molecule to accelerate movement from an area of high concentration to one of low concentration

i. A hormone produced by the adrenal cortex that enhances sodium retention and potassium excretion

j. Process in which molecules move against the concentration gradient; requires energy

k. Any solution with a solute concentration (osmolarity) greater than that of normal body fluids (greater than 310 mOsm/L)

l. The osmotic pressure exerted by colloids in solution; pulls fluid from the tissue space to the vascular space

m. Any solution with a solute concentration (osmolarity) less than that of normal body fluids (less than 270 mOsm/L)

Exercise 2

Virtual Hospital Activity

30 minutes

- Sign in to work at Pacific View Regional Hospital for Period of Care 1. (*Note:* If you are already in the virtual hospital from a previous exercise, click on **Leave the Floor** and then on **Restart the Program** to get to the sign-in window.)
- From the Patient List, select Piya Jordan (Room 403).
- Click on **Go to Nurses' Station**.
- Click on **Chart** and then on **403**.
- Click on **Emergency Department** and **Nursing Admission** and review these records.

1. Record findings below that support the diagnosis of extracellular fluid (ECF) volume deficit.

- Now click on the **Laboratory Reports** tab.

2. Piya Jordan's sodium is elevated at 147 mEq/L. Which of the following manifestations may be noted in the client with hypernatremia and ECF volume deficit? Select all that apply.

_____ Dizziness

_____ Headache

_____ Thirst

_____ Hypertension

_____ ECG changes

_____ Lethargy

_____ Restlessness

- Click on **History and Physical**.

3. What contributing factor(s) led to this fluid imbalance?

- Now click on **Physician's Orders** and read the initial orders for Piya Jordan.

4. Identify orders that are appropriate management strategies for the treatment of ECF volume deficit and write your findings below.

5. Develop an appropriate plan of care for Piya Jordan related to management of her ECF volume deficit.

Collaborative Plan of Care	ECF Volume Deficit
Patient outcomes	
Assessment parameters	
Collaborative care interventions	

Exercise 3

Virtual Hospital Activity

45 minutes

- Sign in to work at Pacific View Regional Hospital for Period of Care 1. (*Note:* If you are already in the virtual hospital from a previous exercise, click on **Leave the Floor** and then on **Restart the Program** to get to the sign-in window.)
- From the Patient List, select Patricia Newman (Room 406).
- Click on **Go to Nurses' Station**.
- Click on **Chart** and then on **406**.
- Click on **Emergency Department** and review the record.
- Click on **Nursing Admission** and review the record.
- Click on **Laboratory Reports** and review test results.

1. Patricia Newman's potassium level is low. A normal potassium level is _____ to

   _____.

2. A potential cause of hypokalemia is:
   a. ACE inhibitors.
   b. acidosis.
   c. vomiting and diarrhea.
   d. renal disease.

3. What clinical manifestations may be noted with hypokalemia? Select all that apply.

_____   Anxiety

_____   Diarrhea

_____   Fatigue

_____   Muscle weakness

_____   Vomiting

_____   Leg cramps

4. Based on your findings, does Patricia Newman have a fluid imbalance? If so, what type?

5. What are the contributing factors for this patient's potential or actual fluid imbalance?

- Read Patricia Newman's **History and Physical**.

6. What coexisting illness might have an impact on the selection and rate of IV fluid therapy?

7. Develop an appropriate plan of care for patients with ECF volume excess by completing the chart below.

Collaborative Plan of Care	ECF Volume Excess
Patient outcomes	
Assessment parameters	
Collaborative care interventions	

Electrolyte Imbalances: Potassium, Calcium, Phosphate, and Sodium

Reading Assignment: Fluid, Electrolyte, and Acid-Base Imbalances (Chapter 16)

Patients: Piya Jordan, Room 403
Pablo Rodriguez, Room 405
Patricia Newman, Room 406

Goal: To utilize the nursing process to competently care for patients with electrolyte imbalances.

Objectives:

1. Describe normal physiologic influences on electrolyte balance.
2. Identify specific etiologic factors related to hypokalemia, hypercalcemia, hyponatremia, and hypophosphatemia for assigned patients.
3. Research potential drug interactions related to hypokalemia for assigned patients.
4. Assess patients for clinical manifestations related to potassium, sodium, calcium, and phosphate imbalances.
5. Utilize the nursing process to correctly administer IV potassium chloride per physician orders.
6. Evaluate the effectiveness of medication prescribed to treat electrolyte imbalances.

In this lesson, you will assess, plan, and implement care for three patients with electrolyte imbalances. Piya Jordan is a 68-year-old female admitted with nausea and vomiting for several days following weeks of poor appetite and increasing weakness. Patricia Newman is a 61-year-old female admitted with pneumonia and a history of emphysema for 12 years. Pablo Rodriguez is a 71-year-old male who is admitted with nausea and vomiting for several days. He has a history of non-small cell lung carcinoma. Begin this activity by reviewing the functions of electrolytes within the body as presented in your textbook. Answer the following questions to cement your understanding of the normal physiologic concepts related to potassium, sodium, calcium, and phosphate balance.

Exercise 1

Writing Activity

20 minutes

1. Below, match each term with its corresponding definition.

Term	Definition
_____ Ion	a. A positively charged ion
_____ Cation	b. The electrical charge of an ion; the degree of combining power of an ion
_____ Anion	c. Electrically charged particle
_____ Valence	d. A negatively charged ion

2. Complete each of the following statements by filling in the blanks.

    a. The primary ICF cation is _____.

    b. The primary ICF anion is _____.

    c. The primary ECF cation is _____.

    d. The primary ECF anion is _____.

3. Identify the functions of potassium within the body. Select all that apply.

    _____ Transmit and conduct nerve impulses

    _____ Maintain normal cardiac rhythms

    _____ Contract skeletal and smooth muscles

    _____ Regulate intracellular osmolality

    _____ Promote cellular growth

    _____ Help maintain acid-base balance

4. Describe the physiologic influences on potassium balance.

5. The factors below can potentially result in either hypokalemia or hyperkalemia. Match each potential cause with its resulting condition.

Potential Cause	Condition
_____ Gastrointestinal losses caused by diarrhea, vomiting, fistulas, nasogastric suction	a. Hypokalemia
	b. Hyperkalemia
_____ Renal losses caused by diuretics, hyperaldosteronism, and/or magnesium depletion	
_____ Excessive potassium intake caused by intravenous potassium-containing drugs and/or potassium-containing salt substitute	
_____ Skin losses caused by diaphoresis	
_____ Shift of potassium out of cells caused by acidosis, tissue catabolism, crush injury, and/or tumor lysis syndrome	
_____ Renal disease	
_____ Dialysis	
_____ Shift of potassium into the cells caused by alkalosis, tissue repair, and increased insulin and epinephrine	
_____ Potassium-sparing diuretics	
_____ Lack of potassium intake	
_____ Adrenal insufficiency	
_____ ACE inhibitors	

Exercise 2

Virtual Hospital Activity

40 minutes

- Sign in to work at Pacific View Regional Hospital for Period of Care 1. (*Note:* If you are already in the virtual hospital from a previous exercise, click on **Leave the Floor** and then on **Restart the Program** to get to the sign-in window.)
- From the Patient List, select Piya Jordan (Room 403).
- Click on **Go to Nurses' Station**.
- Click on **Chart** and then on **403**.
- Click on **Laboratory Reports**.

1. Piya Jordan's initial potassium level on Monday at 2200 was _____ mEq/L

- Click on **Emergency Department** and review this record.

2. Which of the following would be the most likely cause for hypokalemia in this patient?
   a. Prolonged nausea and vomiting
   b. Lack of potassium intake
   c. Constipation
   d. Renal losses

3. The physician has ordered KCl 20 mEq in 250 mL NS to infuse over 2 hours. Is this an appropriate rate of infusion?
   a. No
   b. Yes

4. Which of the following assessments must be completed before administering KCl?
   a. Heart rate
   b. Blood pressure
   c. Bowel sounds
   d. Urinary output

5. What is the maximum recommended infusion rate for KCl on the medical-surgical unit?
   a. 5 mEq/hr
   b. 10 mEq/hr
   c. 15 mEq/hr
   d. 20 mEq/hr

- Click again on **Laboratory Reports**.

6. Piya Jordan's potassium level for Tuesday at 0630 is 3.8 mg/dL. Based on her condition and planned medical interventions, which of the following factors has the greatest potential for causing continued potassium loss?
   a. Lack of oral intake
   b. Continued use of IV analgesics
   c. Loss through skin
   d. Placement of a nasogastric tube

- Click on **Return to Nurses' Station**.
- Click on **403** at the bottom of your screen.
- Click on **Patient Care** and then on **Physical Assessment**. Complete a focused assessment by clicking on the body system categories (yellow buttons) and body system subcategories (green buttons).

7. Document the findings of your physical assessment in the chart below. Put an asterisk next to those manifestations that correlate with hypokalemia.

Areas Assessed	Findings on Physical Examination
Cardiovascular	
Respiratory	
Neuromuscular	
Gastrointestinal	
Renal	

• Click on **Chart** and then on **403**.
• Click on **Physician's Orders** and scroll to review the note on Monday at 2200.

8. What did the physician order in response to Piya Jordan's potassium level on Monday at 2200?

Before administering KCl, you will need to assess Piya Jordan's renal status for adequate urinary output.

- Click on **Return to Room 403**.
- Click on **EPR** and then on **Login**.
- Select **403** from the Patient drop-down menu and **Vital Signs** from the Category drop-down menu. Use the arrows at the bottom of the screen to view previously recorded data.

9. What is Piya Jordan's most recent weight?

- Select **Intake and Output** from the Category drop-down menu.

10. What was Piya Jordan's urinary output from 0000 to 0700 on Wednesday? Based on Piya Jordan's body weight, calculate the minimum urine output necessary to receive the potassium infusion.

Prepare to administer this ordered dose of potassium chloride to Piya Jordan by completing the following steps.

- Click on **Exit EPR**.
- Click on **Medication Room** at the bottom of your screen.
- Click on **IV Storage**.
- Click on the bin labeled **Small Volume** and review the list of available medications.
  (*Note:* You may click on **Review MAR** at any time to verify the correct medication order. Remember to look at the patient name on the MAR to make sure you have the correct patient's record and to click on the correct room number tab within the MAR. Click on **Return to Medication Room** after reviewing the correct MAR.)
- From the list of medications in the bin, select **potassium chloride**. Then click on **Put Medication on Tray** and then on **Close Bin**.
- Click on **View Medication Room**.
- Click on **Preparation**. Select the correct medication to administer; then click on **Prepare**.
- Follow the instructions or answer the questions from the Preparation Wizard. Then click on **Next**.
- Choose the correct patient to administer this medication to. Click on **Finish**.
- You can click on **Review Your Medications** and then on **Return to Medication Room** when ready. From the Medication Room, go directly to Piya Jordan's room by clicking on **403** at the bottom of the screen.

Before administering intravenous medications, the patient's IV site must be assessed.

- Click on **Patient Care** and then on **Physical Assessment**.
- Click on **Upper Extremities** (yellow boxes) and then on **Integumentary** (green boxes) from the system subcategories.

11. Document the IV site assessment findings below. Is it appropriate to administer the IV potassium at this time? What other steps should you take to ensure you have adequately addressed the six rights of medication administration?

- After you have collected the appropriate assessment data and are ready for administration, click on **Medication Administration**.
- Next to Select, click the down arrow and choose **Administer** from the drop-down menu.
- Complete the Administration Wizard and click on **Administer to Patient** when done.
- Check **Yes** when asked whether this drug administration should be documented on the MAR.
- Now click on **MAR** at the top of your screen and then on tab **403**.

12. What are Piya Jordan's scheduled morning medications?

13. Which of the following factors should be assessed before administering the scheduled dose of digoxin to Piya Jordan? Select all that apply.

_____ Potassium level

_____ Sodium level

_____ Heart rate

_____ Blood pressure

_____ Digoxin level

14. Based on your assessment findings for the factors in question 13, should the nurse administer the digoxin at this time? Provide the rationale for your answer.

Now let's see how you did!

- Click on **Leave the Floor** at the bottom of your screen.
- From the Floor Menu, click on **Look at Your Preceptor's Evaluation**.
- Click on **Medication Scorecard**.

15. Disregard the report for the routine scheduled medications, but note below whether or not you correctly administered the potassium chloride. If not, why do you think you were incorrect in administering this drug? According to Table C in this scorecard, what are the appropriate resources that should be used and important assessments that should be completed before administering this medication? Did you utilize and perform them correctly?

Exercise 3

Virtual Hospital Activity

30 minutes

- Sign in to work at Pacific View Regional Hospital for Period of Care 1. (*Note:* If you are already in the virtual hospital from a previous exercise, click on **Leave the Floor** and then on **Restart the Program** to get to the sign-in window.)
- From the Patient List, select Patricia Newman (Room 406).
- Click on **Go to Nurses' Station**.
- Click on **Chart** and then on **406**.
- Click on **Laboratory Reports**.

1. Patricia Newman's initial potassium level was _____ mEq/L this morning.

- Click on **History and Physical**.

2. What would be the most likely cause for hypokalemia in this patient?

- Click on **Physician's Orders**.

3. What did the physician order to treat this electrolyte imbalance?

- Click on **Return to Nurses' Station**.
- Click on **MAR** and then on **406**.

4. What is missing from this order? Where could you verify this missing information?

5. What is the difference between the treatment of hypokalemia for Piya Jordan and that for Patricia Newman? Provide a rationale for the difference.

- Click on **Return to Nurses' Station**.
- Click on **Chart** and then on **406**.
- Click on **Physician's Orders**.

6. Look again at the physician's orders. Is there an order for any follow-up lab work? What is the nurse's responsibility in regard to follow-up lab work? How would you handle this situation?

- Click on **Return to Nurses' Station**.
- Click on **406** at the bottom of the screen.
- Click on **Patient Care** and then on **Nurse-Client Interactions**.
- Select and view the video titled **0740: Evaluation—Response to Care**. (*Note:* Check the virtual clock to see whether enough time has elapsed. You can use the fast-forward feature to advance the time by 2-minute intervals if the video is not yet available. Then click again on **Patient Care** and **Nurse-Client Interactions** to refresh the screen.)

7. Although Patricia Newman is happy that her chest does not hurt like it did, what does she verbalize as a concern? What is the nurse's response to the patient's expressed concern?

8. When evaluating the care of Patricia Newman, for what potential complications of IV potassium therapy would you monitor? (*Hint:* Consult the Drug Guide by clicking on the **Drug** icon in the lower left corner of your screen.)

Exercise 4

Virtual Hospital Activity

30 minutes

1. Before caring for a patient with multiple electrolyte imbalances, it is imperative that you first review and reinforce general concepts related to specific electrolytes. Using the textbook, complete the table below by providing information related to calcium, phosphorus, and sodium. As you proceed through the virtual hospital activities that follow this question, refer to this table to relate textbook knowledge to actual patient care.

Electrolyte	Normal Level	Functions	Major Location	Pathophysiologic Influences
Calcium				
Phosphorus				
Sodium				

- Sign in to work at Pacific View Regional Hospital for Period of Care 1. (*Note:* If you are already in the virtual hospital from a previous exercise, click on **Leave the Floor** and then on **Restart the Program** to get to the sign-in window.)
- From the Patient List, select Pablo Rodriguez (Room 405).
- Click on **Go to Nurses' Station**.
- Click on **Chart** and then on **405**.
- Click on **Laboratory Reports**.

2. Complete the table below by recording Pablo Rodriguez's serum chemistry results. Identify abnormal values by marking as H (for high) or L (for low).

Lab Test	Lab Result Tuesday 2000	Lab Result Wednesday 0730
Sodium		
Potassium		
Calcium		
Phosphorus		
Magnesium		

3. What would be the most likely cause for the hyponatremia noted on admission for this patient?

4. Because GI losses of sodium are accompanied by greater or equal losses of water, explain what causes the lower serum sodium concentration.

- Click on **Return to Nurses' Station**.
- Click on **EPR** and then on **Login**.
- Select **405** from the Patient drop-down menu and **Intake and Output** from the Category drop-down menu.

5. Record the intake and output shift totals for Pablo Rodriguez below.

Shift Totals	Tuesday 2300	Wednesday 0700
Intake		
Output		

6. Based on the above intake and output totals obtained after the patient received IV replacement therapy, what factor(s) may be contributing to the persistent hyponatremia? Explain.

7. What laboratory tests might be helpful to assess for the presence of dehydration? Select all that apply.

_____ Erythrocyte sedimentation rate

_____ Hemoglobin/hematocrit

_____ Serum osmolality

_____ Urine osmolality

_____ Urine specific gravity

_____ Serum glucose level

_____ Blood urea nitrogen

- Click on **Return to Nurses' Station**.
- Click on **405**.
- Click on **Patient Care** and then on **Physical Assessment**.

8. Complete a physical assessment for Pablo Rodriguez, specifically looking for clinical manifestations of hyponatremia. Document your findings in the table below; underline the manifestations that correlate with hyponatremia.

Areas Assessed	Findings on Physical Examination
Cardiovascular	
Respiratory	
Neuromuscular	
Gastrointestinal	

9. What additional clinical manifestations of hyponatremia might you expect to find in other patients with this electrolyte imbalance accompanied by hypovolemia?

Exercise 5

Virtual Hospital Activity

35 minutes

- Sign in to work at Pacific View Regional Hospital for Period of Care 3. (*Note:* If you are already in the virtual hospital from a previous exercise, click on **Leave the Floor** and then on **Restart the Program** to get to the sign-in window.)
- From the Patient List, select Pablo Rodriguez (Room 405).
- Click on **Go to Nurses' Station**.
- Click on **Chart** and then on **405**.
- Click on **History and Physical**.

1. On admission, Pablo Rodriguez presented with two electrolyte imbalances:

   hyper_____ and hypo_____.

2. Pablo Rodriguez's calcium level was _____, and his phosphorus level was

   _____.

3. How does this relate to his calcium level? Explain the pathophysiologic rationale supporting your answer.

4. Which of the following factors might best explain the potential cause for the patient's calcium level?
   a. Malignancy
   b. Lack of dietary intake
   c. Constipation
   d. Side effects of radiation therapy

5. The Emergency Department physician has prescribed pamidronate 90 mg IV to treat the hypercalcemia. How will this help?

6. When administering pamidronate, what baseline nursing assessments are indicated? Select all that apply.

   _____ Oral cavity

   _____ Bowel sounds

   _____ BUN and creatinine

   _____ Electrolytes

   _____ Calcium

- Click on **Return to Nurses' Station**.
- Click on **Kardex** and then on tab **405**.

7. What is the purpose of IV hydration in relation to serum calcium levels?

- Click on **Return to Nurses' Station**.
- Click on **MAR** and then on tab **405**.

8. What medication is scheduled to be administered at 1500? What electrolyte imbalance will this medication correct? Explain your answer.

9. What nursing assessments must be completed before this drug is administered? State your rationale for performing each assessment.

10. After successful treatment of Pablo Rodriguez, the nurse must be aware of the possibility of overcorrecting the electrolyte imbalance. For what clinical manifestations should the nurse monitor this patient in regard to hypocalcemia and hyperphosphatemia?

Acid-Base Imbalance

Reading Assignment: Fluid, Electrolyte, and Acid-Base Imbalances (Chapter 16)
Lower Respiratory Problems (Chapter 27)
Obstructive Pulmonary Diseases (Chapter 28)

Patients: Jacquline Catanazaro, Room 402
Patricia Newman, Room 406

Goal: To utilize the nursing process to competently care for patients with acid-base imbalances.

Objectives:

1. Describe the pathophysiologic basis of acid-base imbalance noted in assigned patients.
2. Identify specific etiologic factor(s) related to respiratory acidosis in the assigned patients.
3. Assess the assigned patients for clinical manifestations related to respiratory acidosis.
4. Describe nursing interventions appropriate when caring for specific patients with respiratory acidosis.
5. Evaluate the effectiveness of medication prescribed to treat acid-base imbalances.

In this lesson, you will assess, plan, and implement care for patients with acid-base imbalances. Jacquline Catanazaro is a 45-year-old female admitted with exacerbation of asthma and schizophrenia. Patricia Newman is a 61-year-old female admitted with pneumonia and a history of emphysema for 12 years. Begin this lesson by reviewing the general concepts of acid-base balance as presented in your textbook.

Exercise 1

Writing Activity

20 minutes

1. Define the following terms.

    a. Acid

    b. Base

    c. pH

2. Describe three methods of acid-base homeostasis by completing the following table.

	Type of Defense	Mechanisms of Action
First Line of Defense: Reacts immediately		
Second Line of Defense: Reacts within minutes		
Third Line of Defense: Takes 2-3 days to respond maximally		

Exercise 2

Virtual Hospital Activity

45 minutes

- Sign in to work at Pacific View Regional Hospital for Period of Care 1. (*Note:* If you are already in the virtual hospital from a previous exercise, click on **Leave the Floor** and then on **Restart the Program** to get to the sign-in window.)
- From the Patient List, select Jacquline Catanazaro (Room 402).
- Click on **Go to Nurses' Station**.
- Click on **Chart** and then on **402**.
- Click on **History and Physical**.

1. Which of the following factors increase Jacquline Catanazaro's risk for an acid base imbalance? Select all that apply.

   _____ History of schizophrenia

   _____ Obesity

   _____ Noncompliance with prescribed asthma medications

   _____ History of asthma

   _____ Chronic back problems

- Click on **Return to Nurses' Station**.
- Click on **402** at the bottom of your screen.
- Click on **Patient Care** and then on **Nurse-Client Interactions**.
- Select and view the video titled **0730: Intervention—Airway**. (*Note:* Check the virtual clock to see whether enough time has elapsed. You can use the fast-forward feature to advance the time by 2-minute intervals if the video is not yet available. Then click again on **Patient Care** and **Nurse-Client Interactions** to refresh the screen.)

2. Based on Jacquline Catanazaro's history, what would you expect to be causing her respiratory distress?

3. What advantages are presented by waiting until the arterial blood gases (ABGs) are drawn to give the patient a nebulizer treatment?

- Click on **Chart** and then on **402**.
- Click on **Laboratory Reports**.

4. What are the results of Jacquline Catanazaro's two most recent ABGs? Record them below.

ABGs	Monday 1030	Wednesday 0730
pH		
PaO$_2$		
PaCO$_2$		
O$_2$ sat		
Bicarb		

5. How would you interpret the results in question 4? Is the acid-base imbalance compensated or uncompensated (fully or partially)? Explain your answer.

6. Because this patient's respiratory difficulties are of an acute nature, what acid-base regulation mechanisms would you expect to be working to compensate for her respiratory acidosis?

7. Based on Jacquline Catanazaro's medical diagnosis, what is the underlying pathophysiologic problem leading to the respiratory acidosis?

- Click on **Return to Room 402**.
- Click on **Patient Care** and then on **Physical Assessment**. Complete a focused assessment by clicking on the body system categories (yellow buttons) and body system subcategories (green buttons).

8. Record the findings from your focused assessment in the table below.

Areas Assessed	Findings on Physical Examination
Neurologic	
Musculoskeletal	
Cardiovascular	
Respiratory	
Integumentary	

9. At the time of this assessment, does this patient have any clinical manifestations of respiratory acidosis? If so, please describe. If not, how do you explain?

- Click on **Take Vital Signs**.

10. What is Jacquline Catanazaro's respiratory rate? How does this correlate with her asthma and respiratory acidosis?

11. If Jacquline Catanazaro's pH were 7.2, her physical assessment might reflect differences. Document the expected clinical manifestations of respiratory acidosis below.

Areas Assessed	Expected Findings on Physical Examination
Neurologic	
Cardiovascular	
Gastrointestinal	
Neuromuscular	
Respiratory	

- Click on **Chart** and then on **402**.
- Click on **Physician's Orders**.

12. Look at the most recent physician's orders. What medication is ordered to treat the respiratory acidosis? What is the medication's underlying mechanism of action to correct the acidosis?

13. Assuming the treatment was effective, provide ABG results that demonstrate normal acid-base balance.

Exercise 3

Virtual Hospital Activity

45 minutes

- Sign in to work at Pacific View Regional Hospital for Period of Care 1. (*Note:* If you are already in the virtual hospital from a previous exercise, click on **Leave the Floor** and then on **Restart the Program** to get to the sign-in window.)
- From the Patient List, select Patricia Newman (Room 406).
- Click on **Go to Nurses' Station**.
- Click on **Chart** and then on **406**.
- Click on **History and Physical**.

1. Review Patricia Newman's history. What findings place her at risk for an acid-base imbalance? Select all that apply.

_____ Advancing age

_____ Tobacco use

_____ Diagnosis of pneumonia

_____ Current body weight

_____ History of emphysema

• Click on **Laboratory Reports**.

2. What are the results of Patricia Newman's two most recent ABG tests? Document your findings below.

ABGs	Tuesday 2300	Wednesday 0500
pH		
PaO_2		
$PaCO_2$		
O_2 sat		
Bicarb		

3. Review the results from Patricia Newman's most recent ABG tests in the preceding question. What inferences can be made from the results? Select all that apply.

_____ Hypoxemia noted on Tuesday

_____ Uncompensated acidosis on Tuesday

_____ Partially compensated acidosis on Wednesday

_____ Normal acid base results on Tuesday

_____ Elevated bicarbonate results on Tuesday

4. Based on the chronic aspect of Patricia Newman's respiratory difficulties, what compensatory mechanisms would you expect to be working to correct the respiratory acidosis?

5. Based on the ABG results, what statement is most accurate concerning Patricia Newman's condition?
   a. She is largely improved.
   b. She is demonstrating a worsening of her condition.
   c. There is little change in her condition.

• Click on **Return to Nurse's Station**.
• Click on **Chart** and then on **406**.
• Click on **Nurse's Notes**.

6. Read the notes for Wednesday at 0730. Describe the actions taken by the nurse. Are they appropriate or not? Explain your answer.

7. What additional actions would be appropriate in the patient's care at this time? Select all that apply.

_____ Maintain oxygen administration

_____ Provide education concerning condition

_____ Lower head of bed

_____ Encourage ambulation

_____ Notify physician

- Click on **Laboratory Reports**.

8. Patricia Newman's serum potassium level is _____ mEq/L on Wednesday at 0500.

9. Hyperkalemia is frequently associated with acidosis as potassium moves out of the cell to compensate for hydrogen moving into the cell. How, then, would you explain the patient's hypokalemia occurring along with respiratory acidosis?

10. Based on Patricia Newman's medical diagnosis, what is the underlying pathophysiologic problem leading to her respiratory acidosis? How does this differ from Jacquline Catanazaro's problem in Exercise 2?

- Click on **Return to Room 406**.
- Click on **Patient Care** and then on **Physical Assessment**. Conduct a physical assessment by clicking on the various body system categories (yellow buttons) and body system subcategories (green buttons).

11. Perform a complete physical assessment, including vital signs, on Patricia Newman. Document your findings below.

Systems Assessed	Findings on Physical Examination
Neurologic	
Musculoskeletal	
Cardiovascular	
Respiratory	
Integumentary	

12. Does Patricia Newman have any clinical manifestations of respiratory acidosis? If so, please describe. If not, explain why not.

13. What nursing interventions could the nurse plan and implement to improve Patricia Newman's acid-base balance and prevent complications?

LESSON **9** _____

Perioperative Care

_____

Reading Assignment: Preoperative Care (Chapter 17)
Postoperative Care (Chapter 19)

Patients: Piya Jordan, Room 403
Clarence Hughes, Room 404

Goal: To utilize the nursing process to competently care for perioperative patients.

Objectives:

1. Document a complete history and physical on a preoperative patient.
2. Identify appropriate rationales for preoperative orders on an assigned patient.
3. Evaluate completeness of preoperative teaching for a patient scheduled for surgery.
4. Document a focused assessment on a patient transferred from a postanesthesia care unit (PACU) to a medical-surgical unit.
5. Plan appropriate interventions to prevent postoperative complications in an assigned patient.
6. Utilize the nursing process to correctly administer scheduled and prn medications to an assigned patient.

In this lesson, you will learn the essentials of caring for patients in both the preoperative and postoperative stages of surgery. You will document, assess, plan, implement, and evaluate care. Piya Jordan is a 68-year-old female admitted with nausea and vomiting for 3 days. Clarence Hughes is a 73-year-old male admitted for an elective knee replacement.

Exercise 1

Virtual Hospital Activity

40 minutes

- Sign in to work at Pacific View Regional Hospital for Period of Care 1. (*Note:* If you are already in the virtual hospital from a previous exercise, click on **Leave the Floor** and then on **Restart the Program** to get to the sign-in window.)
- From the Patient List, select Piya Jordan (Room 403).
- Click on **Go to Nurses' Station**.
- Click on **Chart** and then on **403**.
- Click on **Emergency Department**.

1. On Monday evening Piya Jordan reported to the Emergency Department with complaints of abdominal pain, nausea and vomiting. What were the primary and secondary admitting diagnoses?

- Click on **Nursing Admission**.

2. A review of Piya Jordan's health history and admission data reveals a series of factors that place her at an increased risk for complications. Below, identify the factors that will increase her risk for developing complications. Select all that apply.

_____ Buddhist faith

_____ Obesity

_____ Heart disease

_____ Nutritional imbalance

_____ Age

3. Piya Jordan's admission information indicates that she uses "various herbs," the names of which are not specified. Why is it important to determine the specific therapies being ingested?

- Click on **History and Physical**.

4. In addition to data obtained from the health history, a physical examination provides necessary and important data for the preoperative assessment. For each of the areas listed below and on the next page, identify in the middle column the key items to assess (excluding history and lab results). In the last column, document the results from the physician's assessment as noted in the History and Physical. If an area was not completed, write "No data."

Physical Examination Area	Key Specific Assessments from Textbook	Results for Piya Jordan
Cardiovascular		
Respiratory		
Neurologic		

Physical Examination Area	Key Specific Assessments from Textbook	Results for Piya Jordan
Genitourinary		
Hepatic		
Integumentary		
Musculoskeletal		
Gastrointestinal		

• Click on **Laboratory Reports**.

5. Piya Jordan had lab tests completed before surgery. Record the most recent preoperative results (Mon 2200 and Tue 0630) for the tests below. Access the Lab Guide on the desk of the Nurses' Station. Using the Lab Guide reference values, indicate with an X any results outside normal limits.

Laboratory Test	Most Recent Results	Outside Normal Limits
White blood cell count (WBC)		
Red blood cell count (RBC)		
Hemoglobin		
Hematocrit		
Platelets		
Glucose		
International normalized ratio (INR)		
Sodium		
Potassium		
Blood urea nitrogen (BUN)		
Protein		
Albumin		

6. Review Piya Jordan's lab results again. Which abnormal findings are of concern and need to be addressed before surgery? Explain your answer.

Exercise 2

Virtual Hospital Activity

30 minutes

- Sign in to work at Pacific View Regional Hospital for Period of Care 1. (*Note:* If you are already in the virtual hospital from a previous exercise, click on **Leave the Floor** and then on **Restart the Program** to get to the sign-in window.)
- From the Patient List, select Piya Jordan (Room 403).
- Click on **Go to Nurses' Station**.
- Click on **Chart** and then on **403**.
- Click on the **Consents** tab.

1. For what procedure(s) has Piya Jordan given written consent?

2. Who is responsible for providing detailed information about the procedure(s) for which the patient has given consent?

3. List the three elements that must be present in an informed consent.

4. _____ A signed consent may be revoked at anytime by the patient. (True/False)

5. What are the responsibilities for the nurse concerning the surgical consent? Select all that apply.

_____ Provide a detailed explanation of the procedure to be performed

_____ Witness the patient's signature

_____ Ensure that the patient or responsible party is giving consent voluntarily

_____ Ensure that the patient or responsible party understands the information provided in the consent form

_____ Ensure that the patient and family have a realistic understanding of potential postoperative complications.

• Click on **Physician's Orders**.

6. Look at the orders for Tuesday 0130. What consent was ordered?

7. What is the purpose for the mineral oil enema that was ordered to be given to Piya Jordan?

8. Piya Jordan's surgeon has ordered her to be NPO preoperatively to reduce the risk for aspiration during anesthesia and surgery. It is generally recommended that at least _____ hours pass between the ingestion of a regular diet and a surgical procedure.
   a. 3
   b. 4
   c. 6
   d. 8

9. What is the rationale for giving Piya Jordan a unit of fresh frozen plasma preoperatively?

10. What is the rationale for ordering a dose of cefotetan on call to the operating room? Is this a safe order to administer to Piya Jordan? Explain why or why not.

- Click on **Surgical Reports**.

11. Scroll down to the Preoperative Patient Instruction Sheet. What preoperative teaching was completed?

12. Scroll down further to the Preoperative Checklist. What additional teaching was given to Piya Jordan before admission?

13. What process information should be explained to Piya Jordan's family?

Exercise 3

Virtual Hospital Activity

45 minutes

Clarence Hughes' scheduled surgery is now complete. You will be reviewing care provided to him in the first moments of the postoperative period. Additionally, you will be planning and evaluating care for this current period of care.

- Sign in to work at Pacific View Regional Hospital for Period of Care 1. (*Note:* If you are already in the virtual hospital from a previous exercise, click on **Leave the Floor** and then on **Restart the Program** to get to the sign-in window.)
- From the Patient List, select Clarence Hughes (Room 404).
- Click on **Go to Nurses' Station**.
- Click on **EPR** and then on **Login**.
- Select **404** from the Patient drop-down menu and **Vital Signs** from the Category drop-down menu.
- Use the Category drop-down menu to review other portions of the EPR such as Respiratory, Neurologic, Integumentary, IV, Wounds and Drains, Excretory, and any other EPR categories necessary to answer the following question.

1. On arrival to the medical-surgical clinical unit, a postoperative patient requires an immediate focused assessment. For each area specified in the left column below and on the next page, document the assessment findings recorded by the nurse on Sunday at 1600 when Clarence Hughes arrived on the medical-surgical clinical unit.

Focused Assessment Areas	Clarence Hughes' Assessment Findings
Respiratory	
Neurologic	
Psychologic	
Wound, dressing, and drainage tubes	
Vital signs	
Intravenous fluids	
Color and appearance of skin	
Urinary status	

2. How would you analyze Clarence Hughes' blood pressure and heart rate as recorded in the previous question? What actions should be taken? How often should vital signs be monitored?

3. At what point would you notify the surgeon regarding Clarence Hughes' vital signs?

- Still in the EPR, select **Intake and Output** as the category.

4. In the table below, record Clarence Hughes' intake and output for the past 3 days at the times specified.

	Sun 1500-2300	Mon 2300-0700	Mon 0700-1500	Mon 1500-2300	Tues 2300-0700	Tues 0700-1500	Tues 1500-2300	Wed 2300-0700
Intake								
Output								

5. Is Clarence Hughes' intake or output greater? By how much? Is this expected?

6. What are the possible consequences if this trend in fluid balance continues?

- Click on **Exit EPR**.
- Click on **Chart** and then on **404**.
- Click on **Physician's Orders**.

7. Look at the physician's postoperative orders written on Sunday at 1600. What is ordered to prevent postoperative atelectasis?

8. What additional interventions can you suggest to further prevent atelectasis?

9. What is ordered to prevent deep vein thrombosis (DVT)?

10. Scroll up to look at the orders for Monday 0715. What did the physician order at this time to prevent DVT postoperatively?

11. What additional interventions can you suggest to further prevent DVT?

12. What wound care is ordered on Sunday?

13. Who typically removes the original surgical dressing?

- Click on **Return to Nurse's Station**.
- Click on **404** at the bottom of the screen.
- Click on **Take Vital Signs**. Review these results.
- Next, click on **Clinical Alerts**.
- Click on **Patient Care** and then on **Nurse-Client Interactions**.
- Select and view the video titled **0735: Empathy**. (*Note:* Check the virtual clock to see whether enough time has elapsed. You can use the fast-forward feature to advance the time by 2-minute intervals if the video is not yet available. Then click again on **Patient Care** and **Nurse-Client Interactions** to refresh the screen.)

14. What is Clarence Hughes' major concern at this point?

- Now click on **Medication Room**.
- From the Medication Room, click on **MAR** to determine the medications that have been ordered at 0800 for Clarence Hughes and any appropriate prn medications you may want to administer. (*Note:* You may click on **Review MAR** at any time to verify the correct medication order. Remember to look at the patient name on the MAR to make sure you have the correct patient's record. You must click on the correct room number within the MAR. Click on **Return to Medication Room** after reviewing the correct MAR.)
- Click on **Unit Dosage** at the top of your screen or on the Unit Dosage cabinet to the right of Automated System.
- From the close-up view of the Unit Dosage drawers, click on drawer **404**.
- From the list of available medications in the top window, select the medication(s) you would like to administer. After each medication you select, click on **Put Medication on Tray**.
- When you have finished putting your selected medications on the tray, click on **Close Drawer**.
- Click on **View Medication Room**.
- Click on **Automated System** (or on the Automated System unit itself). Your name and password will automatically appear. Click on **Login**.
- In box 1, select the correct patient; in box 2, choose the appropriate Automated System Drawer for this patient. Then click on **Open Drawer**.

- From the list of available medications, select the medication(s) you would like to administer. For each one selected, click on **Put Medication on Tray**. When you are finished, click on **Close Drawer**.
- Click on **View Medication Room**.
- From the Medication Room, click on **Preparation** (or on the preparation tray on the counter); then highlight the medication you want to administer. Click on **Prepare**.
- Provide any information requested by the Preparation Wizard.
- Click on **Next**, choose the correct patient to administer this medication to, and click on **Finish**.
- Repeat the previous three steps until you have prepared all the medications you want to administer.
- You can click on **Review Your Medications** and then on **Return to Medication Room** when you are ready. Once you are back in the Medication Room, you can go directly to Clarence Hughes' room by clicking on **404** at the bottom of the screen.
- Administer the medication, utilizing the six rights of medication administration. After you have collected the appropriate assessment data and are ready for administration, click on **Patient Care** and then on **Medication Administration**. Verify that the correct patient and medication(s) appear in the left-hand window. Then click the down arrow next to Select. From the drop-down menu, select **Administer** and complete the Administration Wizard by providing any information requested. When the Wizard stops asking for information, click on **Administer to Patient**. Specify **Yes** when asked whether this administration should be recorded in the MAR. Finally, click on **Finish**.

Now let's see how you did!

- Click on **Leave the Floor** at the bottom of your screen.
- From the Floor Menu, select **Look at Your Preceptor's Evaluation**.
- Click on **Medication Scorecard**.

15. Note below whether or not you correctly administered the appropriate medication(s). If not, why do you think you were incorrect? According to Table C in this scorecard, what resources should be used and what important assessments should be completed before administering the medication(s)? Did you utilize these resources and perform these assessments correctly?

Glaucoma

Reading Assignment: Assessment of Visual and Auditory Problems (Chapter 20)
Visual and Auditory Problems (Chapter 21)

Patient: Clarence Hughes, Room 404

Goal: To utilize the nursing process to competently care for patients with glaucoma.

Objectives:

1. Describe the pathophysiology of glaucoma.
2. Identify clinical manifestations related to glaucoma.
3. Describe appropriate pharmacologic treatment of glaucoma.
4. Administer eyedrops safely and accurately.
5. Evaluate a patient's ability to correctly administer prescribed ophthalmic medication.

In this lesson, you will learn the essentials of caring for a patient diagnosed with glaucoma. You will explore the patient's history, evaluate presenting symptoms and treatment, administer prescribed medications, and develop an individualized discharge teaching plan. Clarence Hughes is a 73-year-old male admitted for an elective left knee arthroplasty.

Exercise 1

Writing Activity

15 minutes

1. Briefly describe the general pathophysiology of glaucoma.

2. Which of the following statements regarding glaucoma is correct? Select all that apply.

_____ Glaucoma is characterized by decreased intraocular pressure (IOP).

_____ Visual changes that result from glaucoma can be successfully cured with laser therapies.

_____ The incidence of glaucoma among African-Americans is greater than in Caucasians.

_____ Typically, central vision is the first visual loss associated with glaucoma.

_____ Normal IOP is 10 to 21 mm Hg.

_____ Miotic medications may be used to reduce IOP.

3. Compare and contrast the three different types of glaucoma by completing the following table.

Type of Glaucoma	Etiology	Pathophysiology	Clinical Manifestations
Primary open-angle			
Primary angle-closure			

4. Identify and describe the measures used to diagnose glaucoma.

Exercise 2

Virtual Hospital Activity

45 minutes

- Sign in to work at Pacific View Regional Hospital for Period of Care 3. (*Note:* If you are already in the virtual hospital from a previous exercise, click on **Leave the Floor** and then on **Restart the Program** to get to the sign-in window.)
- From the Patient List, select Clarence Hughes (Room 404).
- Click on **Go to Nurses' Station**.
- Click on **Chart** and then on **404**.
- Click on **History and Physical**.

1. What problem of the eye does Clarence Hughes have?

2. How would this be diagnosed?

3. Primary open angle glaucoma (PAOG) is traditionally silent in the early stages. Which of the following symptoms, when noted, may be present with glaucoma?
   a. Eye pain
   b. Peripheral vision loss
   c. Seeing colored halos around lights
   d. Nausea

4. The History and Physical does not identify the type of glaucoma Clarence Hughes has. Based on his history and information in your textbook, which type do you think he most likely has? Explain why you came to this conclusion.

- Click on **Return to Nurses' Station**.
- Click on **MAR** and then on tab **404**.

5. What medications are ordered for Clarence Hughes' glaucoma? Identify these medications, their classifications, and mechanisms of action in the first three columns of the table below. (*Note:* You will complete the last column in question 7.)

Medication	Drug Classification	Mechanism of Action	Side Effects

6. For what side effects related to these medications should you monitor Clarence Hughes? Record your answer in the table above.

- Click on **Return to Nurses' Station**.
- Click on the **Drug** icon in the lower left corner of the screen to access the Drug Guide.
- Use the Search box or scroll to find the medications ordered for Clarence Hughes' glaucoma.

7. If you were to administer the prescribed antiglaucoma medications to Clarence Hughes, how would you correctly apply the eye drops? Explain the step-by-step procedure described in the Drug Guide.

- Click on **Return to Nurses' Station**.
- Click on **Chart** and then on **404**.
- Click on **Patient Education**.

8. What educational goals would you add for Clarence Hughes related to his glaucoma?

9. What teaching would you provide for this patient regarding his glaucoma?

10. Which of the following teaching points should be included in the patient education when discussing the use of timolol maleate to manage Clarence Hughes' condition? Select all that apply.

_____ Do not abruptly discontinue use

_____ Report feelings of excessive fatigue

_____ Avoid use of over-the-counter medications without physician's approval

_____ Drink several glasses of water each day

_____ Nighttime visual changes may result with medication

_____ Avoid alcohol intake

_____ Limit salt intake

_____ Report stinging or discomfort if experienced with instillation of medication

11. What methods would you use to teach medication administration to this patient?

12. How would you evaluate Clarence Hughes' understanding of correct medication application?

13. If Clarence Hughes' ophthalmic medications would fail to maintain IOP within normal limits, what other therapies might he expect to undergo? Briefly describe each procedure.

LESSON 11 ————————————————

Chronic Obstructive Pulmonary Disease and Pneumonia

Reading Assignment: Lower Respiratory Problems (Chapter 27)
Obstructive Pulmonary Diseases (Chapter 28)

Patient: Patricia Newman, Room 406

Goal: To utilize the nursing process to competently care for patients with altered oxygenation states.

Objectives:

1. Relate physical assessment findings with pathophysiologic changes of the lower respiratory tract.
2. Prioritize nursing care for a patient with altered oxygenation.
3. Evaluate laboratory results relative to the diagnosis of pneumonia and chronic obstructive pulmonary disease (COPD).
4. Describe pharmacologic interventions related to altered oxygenation states.
5. Identify appropriate nursing interventions for a patient admitted with pneumonia and COPD.
6. Identify appropriate discharge teaching needs for a patient with altered oxygenation.

In this lesson, you will learn the essentials of caring for a patient diagnosed with pneumonia and COPD. You will explore the patient's history, evaluate presenting symptoms and treatment on admission, and assess the patient's progress throughout the hospital stay. Patricia Newman is a 61-year-old female admitted with pneumonia and a history of COPD. Begin this lesson by reviewing the general concepts of COPD and pneumonia as presented in your textbook.

Exercise 1

Writing Activity

10 minutes

1. Describe the pathophysiology of chronic obstructive pulmonary disease (COPD).

2. Which of the following statements concerning COPD is correct?
   a. Early diagnosis of the condition will allow for the patient to make a full recovery with curative medication therapies.
   b. The condition is characterized by inflammation of the upper airways resulting in a chronic cough and wheezing.
   c. Inflammation of the lower airways develops after exposure to a bacterial or viral irritant.
   d. Bronchioles lose their shape and become clogged with mucus, and walls of alveoli are destroyed, resulting in fewer alveoli for gas exchange.

3. Pneumonia consists of four characteristic stages. Match each stage with its corresponding characteristics.

Stage	**Characteristics**
_____ Stage 1: Congestion	a. Massive dilation of capillaries; alveoli fill with organisms, neutrophils, red blood cells, and fibrin.
_____ Stage 2: Red hepatization	
	b. Leukocytes and fibrin consolidate in the affected part of the lungs.
_____ Stage 3: Gray hepatization	
_____ Stage 4: Resolution	c. Exudate is lysed and processed by the macrophages.
	d. The alveoli receive an outpouring of fluid. Organisms multiply in the serous fluid spreading infection to adjacent alveoli.

4. Identify factors that may increase a patient's risk for developing pneumonia.

Exercise 2

Virtual Hospital Activity

45 minutes

- Sign in to work at Pacific View Regional Hospital for Period of Care 1. (*Note:* If you are already in the virtual hospital from a previous exercise, click on **Leave the Floor** and then on **Restart the Program** to get to the sign-in window.)
- From the Patient List, select Patricia Newman (Room 406).
- Click on **Get Report**.

1. What questions would you ask the outgoing nurses to obtain needed information not identified in report?

2. Below, relate the clinical manifestations identified in the change-of-shift report to the patient's diagnosis of pneumonia.

Clinical Manifestations	Pathophysiologic Basis
Labored respirations	
Use of accessory muscles	
Productive cough with yellow sputum	
Coarse breath sounds	
Lung infiltrates	
Disturbed sleep patterns	
Tachycardia	
Fever	

- Click on **Go to Nurses' Station**.
- Click on **Chart** and then on **406**.
- Click on **History and Physical**.

3. What risk factors for community-acquired pneumonia does Patricia Newman have?

- Click on **Return to Nurses' Station**.
- Click on **406** at the bottom of your screen.
- Read the Initial Observations.

4. Each of the following are priority nursing assessments/interventions for Patricia Newman as a result of her current condition. Which action should have the greatest priority?
   a. Assessing vital signs
   b. Auscultating lung sounds
   c. Applying oxygen via nasal cannula at 2 L
   d. Discussing the importance of keeping oxygen on

- Click on **Patient Care** and then on **Physical Assessment**.
- Perform a focused assessment based on Patricia Newman's admitting diagnosis by clicking on the body system categories (yellow buttons) and body system subcategories (green buttons).
- Click on **Nurse-Client Interactions**.
- Select and view the video titled **0730: Prioritizing Interventions**. (*Note:* Check the virtual clock to see whether enough time has elapsed. You can use the fast-forward feature to advance the time by 2-minute intervals if the video is not yet available. Then click again on **Patient Care** and **Nurse-Client Interactions** to refresh the screen.)

5. What nursing interventions would be appropriate to improve Patricia Newman's airway clearance and breathing pattern?

- Click on **Chart** and then on **406**.
- Click on **Laboratory Reports**.

6. Identify any abnormal lab results and describe how they correlate with Patricia Newman's diagnosis of pneumonia.

- Click on **Return to Room 406**.
- Click on **MAR** and then on tab **406**.

7. What is the desired therapeutic effect of ipratropium bromide? How could the nurse assess whether the desired effect was achieved?

8. What is the desired therapeutic effect of cefotetan? How could the nurse assess whether the desired effect was achieved?

9. What is the rationale for administration of IV fluids as related to pneumonia?

• Click on **Return to Room 406**.
• Click on **Medication Room**.
• Click on **MAR** to determine medications that Patricia Newman is ordered to receive at 0800 and any appropriate prn medications you may want to administer. (*Note:* You may click on **Review MAR** at any time to verify the correct medication order. Remember to look at the patient name on the MAR to make sure you have the correct patient's record and to click on the correct room number within the MAR. Click on **Return to Medication Room** after reviewing the correct MAR.)
• Click on **Unit Dosage**. When the close-up view appears, click on drawer **406**.
• Select the medication(s) you plan to administer. After each medication you select, click on **Put Medication on Tray**. When you are finished, click on **Close Drawer**.
• Click on **View Medication Room**.
• Click on **IV Storage**. From the close-up view, click on the drawer labeled **Large Volume**.
• Select the medication(s) you plan to administer, put the medication(s) on the tray, and close the bin.
• Click on **View Medication Room**.
• Click on **Preparation**. Select the correct medication to administer.
• Click on **Prepare** and then on **Next.**
• Choose the correct patient to administer this medication to and click on **Finish.**
• Repeat the above three steps until all medications that you want to administer are prepared.
• You can click on **Review Your Medications** and then on **Return to Medication Room** when ready. From the Medication Room, you can go directly to Patricia Newman's room by clicking on **406** at the bottom of the screen.

- Administer the medication utilizing the six rights of medication administration. After you have collected the appropriate assessment data and are ready for administration, click on **Patient Care** and then on **Medication Administration**. Verify that the correct patient and medication(s) appear in the left-hand window. Then click the down arrow next to Select. From the drop-down menu, select **Administer** and complete the Administration Wizard by providing any information requested. When the Wizard stops asking for information, click on **Administer to Patient**. Specify **Yes** when asked whether this administration should be recorded in the MAR. Finally, click on **Finish**.

Now let's see how you did!

- Click on **Leave the Floor** at the bottom of your screen.
- From the Floor Menu, select **Look at Your Preceptor's Evaluation**.
- Click on **Medication Scorecard**.

10. Note below whether or not you correctly administered the appropriate medications. If not, why do you think you were incorrect? According to Table C in this scorecard, what are the appropriate resources that should be used and important assessments that should be completed before administering these medications? Did you use these resources and perform these assessments correctly?

Exercise 3

Virtual Hospital Activity

40 minutes

- Sign in to work at Pacific View Regional Hospital for Period of Care 2. (*Note:* If you are already in the virtual hospital from a previous exercise, click on **Leave the Floor** and then on **Restart the Program** to get to the sign-in window.)
- From the Patient List, select Patricia Newman (Room 406).
- Click on **Go to Nurses' Station**.
- Click on **Chart** and then on **406**.
- Click on **History and Physical**.

1. How long has Patricia Newman been diagnosed with COPD?

2. What clinical manifestations documented on the History and Physical can be attributed to COPD?

3. What additional clinical manifestations might you expect to see in other patients with COPD?

- Click on **Diagnostic Reports**.

4. What findings on the chest x-ray are consistent with the diagnosis of COPD?

5. What is the relationship between the patient's admitting diagnosis (pneumonia) and her underlying chronic lung condition (COPD)?

- Click on **Physician's Orders**.

6. What is the order for oxygen?

- Click on **Patient Education**.

7. What is educational goal 3 for Patricia Newman?

8. Pursed-lip breathing is a goal for Patricia Newman. When providing education for the technique, which of the following instructions should be included? Select all that apply.

_____ Perform pursed-lip breathing during any activity that causes shortness of breath.

_____ Pursed-lip breathing is most effective when performed while standing.

_____ Leaning forward while sitting is an effective position in which to perform pursed-lip breathing.

_____ When exhaling during pursed-lip breathing, the cheeks should be puffed.

_____ Inhale through the nose during pursed-lip breathing.

9. What is educational goal 4 for Patricia Newman?

10. Patricia Newman is underweight. Weight loss is commonly associated with COPD. Which of the following factors are associated with this manifestation? Select all that apply.

_____ Poor appetite

_____ Decreased energy consumption

_____ Gastric distention pressing on the diaphragm

_____ Shortness of breath

_____ Swallowing air while eating

11. When planning the diet for Patricia Newman, which of the following recommendations should be made?
a. The patient will need at least 4 liters of fluid intake each day.
b. The patient should consume a low-protein, high-carbohydrate diet.
c. The patient should consume 1% milk to aid in mucus control.
d. The patient should schedule treatments about 30 minutes before meals.

12. Demonstration of effective coughing technique is an educational goal for Patricia Newman. Explain the rationale for using the effective huff coughing technique. How would you teach this patient to cough effectively?

13. Because Patricia Newman's COPD puts her at high risk for pulmonary infections, what would you teach her to do to help prevent further episodes of pneumonia?

• Click on **Return to Nurses' Station**.
• Click on **406** to go to Patricia Newman's room.
• Click on **Patient Care** and then on **Nurse-Client Interactions**.
• Select and view the video titled **1100: Care Coordination**. (*Note:* Check the virtual clock to see whether enough time has elapsed. You can use the fast-forward feature to advance the time by 2-minute intervals if the video is not yet available. Then click again on **Patient Care** and **Nurse-Client Interactions** to refresh the screen.)

14. What disciplines are involved in planning and providing care for Patricia Newman? List these in the left column below. In the right column, explain the role of each person in helping meet the patient's health care needs.

Involved Disciplines   **Role in Patricia Newman's Health Care**

LESSON 12

Asthma

Reading Assignment: Assessment of Respiratory System (Chapter 25)
Obstructive Pulmonary Diseases (Chapter 28)

Patient: Jacquline Catanazaro, Room 402

Goal: To utilize the nursing process to competently care for patients with asthma.

Objectives:

1. Identify clinical manifestations of an acute asthmatic exacerbation.
2. Evaluate diagnostic tests as they relate to a patient's oxygenation status.
3. Describe medications used to treat asthma, including mechanism of action and therapeutic effects.
4. Prioritize nursing care for a patient with an acute exacerbation of asthma.
5. Formulate an appropriate patient education plan regarding home asthma management for a patient with identified barriers to learning.

In this lesson, you will learn the essentials of caring for a patient diagnosed with asthma. You will explore the patient's history, evaluate presenting symptoms and treatment on admission, and follow the patient's progress throughout the hospital stay. Jacquline Catanazaro is a 45-year-old female admitted with increasing respiratory distress. Begin this lesson by reviewing the general concepts of asthma as presented in your textbook.

Exercise 1

Writing Activity

20 minutes

1. Briefly describe the pathophysiology of asthma.

2. Match each asthma classification with its corresponding clinical features.

Classification	Characteristics
_____ Intermittent	a. Symptoms occur daily. Nighttime awakening occurs more than once per week, but not daily. Daily use of inhaled short-acting beta$_2$ agonist.
_____ Mild persistent	
_____ Moderate persistent	b. Symptoms occur less than or equal to two times per week. Nighttime awakening less than or equal to twice a month. Symptoms do not interfere with normal activity.
_____ Severe persistent	
	c. Symptoms occur more than two times per week. Symptoms are present at night three or four times a month. Exacerbations may affect activity.
	d. Symptoms are continuously present and cause awakening each night. Short-acting bronchodilator is used multiple times a day. Physical activity is extremely limited by condition.

3. Match each description with the corresponding pulmonary function test (spirometry) result.

Pulmonary Function Test

_____ Forced vital capacity (FVC)

_____ Forced expiratory volume in the second (FEV_1)

_____ Peak expiratory flow rate (PEFR)

Description

a. The amount of air exhaled in the first second of FVC; used to grade the severity of airway obstruction

b. The maximum airflow rate during forced expiration; aids in monitoring bronchoconstriction in asthma; can be measured with peak flow meter

c. The amount of air that can be quickly and forcefully exhaled after maximum inspiration

Exercise 2

Virtual Hospital Activity

40 minutes

- Sign in to work at Pacific View Regional Hospital for Period of Care 1. (*Note:* If you are already in the virtual hospital from a previous exercise, click on **Leave the Floor** and then on **Restart the Program** to get to the sign-in window.)
- From the Patient List, select Jacquline Catanazaro (Room 402).
- Click on **Go to Nurses' Station**.
- Click on **Chart** and then on **402**.
- Click on **History and Physical**.

1. What medical problems does Jacquline Catanazaro have?

2. What pathologic triggers can lead to an exacerbation of asthma?

3. Discuss the potential relationship between Jacquline Catanazaro's schizophrenia and her exacerbation of asthma.

4. Which of the following classifications of asthma best describes Jacquline Catanazaro's condition?
   a. Mild intermittent
   b. Mild persistent
   c. Moderate persistent
   d. Severe persistent

- Click on **Emergency Department**.

5. What were Jacquline Catanazaro's presenting symptoms?

- Click on **Physician's Orders** and review the Emergency Department orders.
- Click on **Laboratory Reports** and review the results for Monday 1030.

6. What diagnostic tests were ordered? Document and interpret the abnormal results below.

- Click on **Emergency Department** and read the note for Monday 1400.

7. What are the results of Jacquline Catanazaro's peak expiratory flow rate (PEFR)? Her predicted PEFR is greater than 200 L/min. How would you interpret these in light of her present condition?

• Click on **Physician's Orders** again and read the orders for Monday 1005.

8. What medical treatments were ordered in the Emergency Department?

9. How would you evaluate the patient's response to medical treatment?

10. Each of the medications below have been ordered for Jacquline Catanazaro. Match each medication with its corresponding action.

Medication	Action
_____ Beclomethasone	a. Promotes bronchodilation and decreases mucosal secretions
_____ Albuterol	b. Inhibits bronchoconstriction, produces smooth muscle relaxation and decreases mucous production
_____ Ipratropium	c. Stimulates beta$_2$ receptors in the lungs, causing relaxation of bronchial smooth muscle

11. _____ The ordered medications listed in the previous question should ideally be administered in a specific order. (True/False)

12. What new medications are ordered on Tuesday at 0800? Give a rationale for these orders. Why is the prednisone ordered to be decreased by 5 mg every day?

Exercise 3

Virtual Hospital Activity

30 minutes

- Sign in to work at Pacific View Regional Hospital for Period of Care 1. (*Note:* If you are already in the virtual hospital from a previous exercise, click on **Leave the Floor** and then on **Restart the Program** to get to the sign-in window.)
- From the Patient List, select Jacquline Catanazaro (Room 402).
- Click on **Go to Nurses' Station**.
- Click on **402** at the bottom of your screen.
- Inside the patient's room, read the Initial Observations.

  1. Describe your initial observations when you enter Jacquline Catanazaro's room.

- Click on **Take Vital Signs**.

  2. Record the patient's vital signs below.

- Click on **Clinical Alerts**.

  3. Are there any clinical alerts for Jacquline Catanazaro? If so, describe below.

  4. How would you prioritize your care for her at this point?

- Click on **Patient Care** and then on **Physical Assessment**.
- Perform a focused assessment by clicking on the body system categories (yellow buttons) and body system subcategories (green buttons).

5. Record the findings from your focused assessment in the table below.

**Focused Areas
of Assessment**   **Jacquline Catanazaro's Assessment Findings**

- Click on **Chart** and then on **402**.
- Click on **Physician's Orders**.

6. What new orders did the physician write on Monday at 0730?

- Click on **Return to Room 402**.
- Click on **Patient Care** and then on **Nurse-Client Interactions**.
- Select and view the video titled **0730: Intervention—Airway**. (*Note:* Check the virtual clock to see whether enough time has elapsed. You can use the fast-forward feature to advance the time by 2-minute intervals if the video is not yet available. Then click again on **Patient Care** and **Nurse-Client Interactions** to refresh the screen.)

7. How does this nurse prioritize her actions? Explain the rationale behind her actions. Is this appropriate?

- Click on **Clinical Alerts**. (*Note:* Check the virtual clock to see whether enough time has elapsed. You can use the fast-forward feature to advance the time by 2-minute intervals if the alert is not yet available. Then click again on **Patient Care** and **Clinical Alerts** to refresh the screen.)

8. Look at the 0800 clinical alert. Interpret this alert below.

- Click on **Chart** and then on **402**.
- Click on **Physician's Orders**. Find the orders for 0800 on Wednesday.

9. Record the orders below and provide a rationale for each.

New Orders	Rationale/Expected Therapeutic Response

10. What objective, noninvasive method might be useful to determine the effectiveness of treatment for Jacquline Catanazaro's acute asthma? Explain.

Exercise 4

Virtual Hospital Activity

45 minutes

- Sign in to work at Pacific View Regional Hospital for Period of Care 2. (*Note:* If you are already in the virtual hospital from a previous exercise, click on **Leave the Floor** and then on **Restart the Program** to get to the sign-in window.)
- From the Patient List, select Jacquline Catanazaro (Room 402).
- Click on **Get Report**.

1. Briefly summarize the activity for Jacquline Catanazaro over the last four hours.

- Click on **Go to Nurses' Station**.
- Click on **402** at the bottom of your screen.

2. What is your initial observation of Jacquline Catanazaro for this time period?

- Click on **Take Vital Signs**.

3. Record Jacquline Catanazaro's current vital signs below. Review your response in Exercise 3, question 2 of this lesson. How do these results compare with those you obtained during Period of Care 1?

- Click on **Patient Care** and then on **Physical Assessment**.
- Perform a focused assessment by clicking on the body system categories (yellow buttons) and body system subcategories (green buttons).

4. Record the findings of your focused assessment in the middle column below. In the right-hand column, compare these findings with the assessment you completed during Period of Care 1 and interpret your results.

Focused Areas of Assessment	Current Findings	Comparison with 0800 Findings—Interpretation of Results (Exercise 3, Question 5)

- Click on **Nurse-Client Interactions**.
- Select and view the video titled **1115: Assessment—Readiness to Learn**. (*Note:* Check the virtual clock to see whether enough time has elapsed. You can use the fast-forward feature to advance the time by 2-minute intervals if the video is not yet available. Then click again on **Patient Care** and **Nurse-Client Interactions** to refresh the screen.)

5. Describe the nurse's actions. Are they appropriate? Explain.

6. What barriers to learning might be present for Jacquline Catanazaro?

- Click on **Chart** and then on **402**.
- Click on **Patient Education**.

7. What are the educational goals for Jacquline Catanazaro?

8. What other asthma management needs would you teach this patient?

9. The patient is scheduled for discharge tomorrow. Do you have any concerns? What would be your most appropriate action?

- Click on **Return to Room 402**.
- Click on **Leave the Floor**.
- Click on **Restart the Program**.
- Sign in to work at Pacific View Regional Hospital for Period of Care 3.
- From the Patient List, select Jacquline Catanazaro (Room 402).
- Click on **Go to Nurses' Station**.
- Click on **402** at the bottom of your screen.
- Click on **Patient Care** and then on **Nurse-Client Interactions**.
- Select and view the video titled **1500: Intervention—Patient Teaching**. (*Note:* Check the virtual clock to see whether enough time has elapsed. You can use the fast-forward feature to advance the time by 2-minute intervals if the video is not yet available. Then click again on **Patient Care** and **Nurse-Client Interactions** to refresh the screen.)

10. What equipment is the nurse teaching Jacquline Catanazaro about?

11. Review your textbook and describe proper use of the peak flow meter for this patient.

12. When providing instruction to a patient about the use of a metered-dose inhaler (MDI), what information should be included? Select all that apply.

_____ Avoid moisture in the care and maintenance of the inhaler device

_____ Shake well before use

_____ Avoid use of spacers with the device

_____ Breathe in slowly with use

_____ Breathe out rapidly with use

Blood Component Therapy

Reading Assignment: Assessment of Hematologic System (Chapter 29)
Hematologic Problems (Chapter 30)

Patient: Piya Jordan, Room 403

Goal: To utilize the nursing process to competently care for patients receiving various blood products.

Objectives:

1. Describe the ABO and Rh antigen systems.
2. Identify the correct type of blood to administer to a specific patient.
3. Describe appropriate nursing responsibilities related to blood product administration.
4. Evaluate vital sign assessments related to potential blood transfusion reactions.
5. Describe appropriate assessment parameters when monitoring for various types of transfusion reactions.

In this lesson, you will learn the essentials of caring for a patient receiving blood and blood product transfusions. You will describe pretransfusion responsibilities, identify administration specifics, and evaluate the patient during and after each transfusion. Piya Jordan is a 68-year-old female admitted with nausea, vomiting, and abdominal pain.

Exercise 1

Writing Activity

15 minutes

1. Describe the ABO antigen system.

2. Describe the Rh antigen system.

3. Complete the table below to identify which types of blood are compatible with each other.

Patient's Blood Type	Blood Types Patient Can Receive
A+	
A−	
B+	
B−	
O+	
O−	
AB+	
AB−	

Exercise 2

Virtual Hospital Activity

30 minutes

- Sign in to work at Pacific View Regional Hospital for Period of Care 1. (*Note:* If you are already in the virtual hospital from a previous exercise, click on **Leave the Floor** and then on **Restart the Program** to get to the sign-in window.)
- From the Patient List, select Piya Jordan (Room 403).
- Click on **Go to Nurses' Station**.
- Click on **Chart** and then on **403**.
- Click on **Laboratory Reports**.

1. Document the results of Piya Jordan's hematology results below.

	Monday 2200	**Tuesday 0630**	**Wednesday 0630**
Hemoglobin			
Hematocrit			

- Click on **Physician's Notes** and review the note for Tuesday at 1730.

2. Why do you think her hemoglobin and hematocrit results are lower on Wednesday?

- Click on **Physician's Orders**.

3. What was ordered to correct this? Is this appropriate related to Piya Jordan's level of hemoglobin? Explain why or why not.

4. The administration of a unit of packed red blood cells can raise the hemoglobin level by _____ g/dL.

The hematocrit level can be raised by _____%.

- Click on **Return to Nurses' Station**.
- Click on **403** at the bottom of your screen.
- Click on **Patient Care** and then on **Nurse-Client Interactions**.
- Select and view the video titled **0735: Pain—Adverse Drug Event**. (*Note:* Check the virtual clock to see whether enough time has elapsed. You can use the fast-forward feature to advance the time by 2-minute intervals if the video is not yet available. Then click again on **Patient Care** and **Nurse-Client Interactions** to refresh the screen.)

5. What does the nurse state she will do to prepare the patient for a blood transfusion?

6. When planning the equipment needed for the IV insertion to transfuse the blood, what would be the minimum needle size necessary?
   a. 24-gauge
   b. 22-gauge
   c. 20-gauge
   d. 18-gauge

7. What other pretransfusion responsibilities would you complete? Have these been completed?

- Click on **Chart** and then on **403**.
- Click on **Laboratory Reports**.

8. _____ is done to verify the compatibility of the donor's blood with the recipient's blood.

9. When preparing the IV to prime the blood tubing, which of the following fluids should be utilized?
   a. Isotonic saline
   b. Lactated Ringer's
   c. 5% dextrose in water
   d. 5% dextrose in lactated Ringer's

Exercise 3

Virtual Hospital Activity

20 minutes

- Sign in to work at Pacific View Regional Hospital for Period of Care 2. (*Note:* If you are already in the virtual hospital from a previous exercise, click on **Leave the Floor** and then on **Restart the Program** to get to the sign-in window.)
- From the Patient List, select Piya Jordan (Room 403).
- Click on **Go to Nurses' Station** and then on **403** at the bottom of your screen.
- Click on **Patient Care** and then on **Nurse-Client Interactions**.
- Select and view the video titled **1115: Interventions—Nausea and Blood**. (*Note:* Check the virtual clock to see whether enough time has elapsed. You can use the fast-forward feature to advance the time by 2-minute intervals if the video is not yet available. Then click again on **Patient Care** and **Nurse-Client Interactions** to refresh the screen.)

1. Piya Jordan's daughter verbalizes concern regarding the safety of blood transfusions. Describe information that should be provided to explain the safety of blood transfusions.

2. During the video, the nurse states that the blood has just arrived. How soon should the nurse begin the transfusion?

- Click on **Chart** and then on **403**.
- Click on **Laboratory Reports**.

3. Piya Jordan has A+ blood. Which type(s) of blood may she receive safely? Select all that apply.

_____ A+

_____ A–

_____ B–

_____ B+

_____ O+

_____ O–

4. What baseline assessment is necessary to complete before beginning the blood transfusion?

5. During the initial period of the transfusion, a nurse recognizes that the rate of infusion should not exceed:
   a. 2 mL/min.
   b. 5 mL/min.
   c. 10 mL/min.
   d. 12 mL/min.

6. When planning care, a nurse must remember that the transfusion of a unit of packed red blood cells must be infused within:
   a. 1 hour.
   b. 2 hours.
   c. 4 hours.
   d. 6 hours.

7. What assessments should be completed on Piya Jordan during the transfusion?

8. What would you document regarding this blood transfusion?

Exercise 4

Virtual Hospital Activity

40 minutes

- Sign in to work at Pacific View Regional Hospital for Period of Care 4. (*Note:* If you are already in the virtual hospital from a previous exercise, click on **Leave the Floor** and then on **Restart the Program** to get to the sign-in window.)
- Click on **EPR** and then on **Login**. (*Remember:* You are not able to visit patients or administer medications during Period of Care 4. You are able to review patients' records only.)
- Select **403** from the Patient drop-down menu and **Vital Signs** from the Category drop-down menu.

1. Review Piya Jordan's vital signs. Did Piya Jordan have any adverse reactions to the blood transfusions? Explain.

2. What symptoms would be anticipated if a hemolytic transfusion resulted? Select all that apply.

_____   Hypothermia

_____   Fever

_____   Diaphoresis

_____   Chills

_____   Low back pain

_____   Bradycardia

_____   Tachypnea

_____   Hypotension

_____   Cloudy urine

3. How would these symptoms differ if she had an allergic transfusion reaction?

4. How can you determine that Piya Jordan did not have a febrile reaction if she was febrile at the beginning of the transfusion?

5. If Piya Jordan would have demonstrated clinical manifestations indicative of a blood transfusion reaction, what nursing interventions would have been appropriate to implement?

• Select **Intake and Output** from the Category drop-down menu. Use the arrows at the bottom of the screen to view previously recorded data.

6. What was Piya Jordan's total intake and output over the last 24 hours (i.e., Tuesday at 1500 through Wednesday at 1500)?

- Click on **Exit EPR**.
- Click on **MAR** and then on tab **403**.

7. Over what period of time was the first unit of red blood cells infused? Was this appropriate? Explain.

8. What signs or symptoms would you expect to see if Piya Jordan was suffering from circulatory overload?

- Click on **Return to Nurses' Station**.
- Click on **Chart** and then on **403**.
- Click on **Expired MARs**.
- Review Tuesday's MAR.

9. What other blood product has she received this admission?

10. How does this product differ from red blood cells? Check the History and Physical to determine why it was given to Piya Jordan.

11. How does administration of fresh frozen plasma differ from administration of red blood cells?

LESSON 14

Hypertension

Reading Assignment: Hypertension (Chapter 32)

Patients: Harry George, Room 401
Patricia Newman, Room 406

Goal: To utilize the nursing process to competently care for patients with hypertension.

Objectives:

1. Describe the classifications of blood pressure.
2. Identify the presence of risk factors for hypertension in assigned patients.
3. Discuss pharmacologic therapies available to treat hypertension.
4. Perform appropriate assessments before administering pharmacologic therapy for hypertension.
5. Develop an extensive educational plan for patients with hypertension.

In this lesson, you will learn the essentials of caring for patients with hypertension. You will explore each patient's history, evaluate presenting symptoms and treatment, identify blood pressure classification, provide appropriate nursing interventions, and plan an appropriate patient education plan related to the hypertension. Patricia Newman is a 61-year-old Caucasian female admitted with pneumonia and a history of emphysema. Harry George is a 54-year-old Caucasian male admitted with infection and swelling of the left foot.

Exercise 1

Writing Activity

20 minutes

1. Identify four categories of blood pressure and the associated blood pressure measurements that define each category.

2. In the table below, identify and describe four physiologic controls of blood pressure.

Physiologic Control	Description

3. Define the following terms.

a. Primary (essential or idiopathic) hypertension

b. Secondary hypertension

4. Which are considered to be risk factors for primary hypertension? Select all that apply.

_____ Advancing age

_____ Slender build

_____ Diabetes mellitus

_____ African American ethnicity

_____ Excessive alcohol use

_____ Family history

_____ Smoking tobacco

5. Listed below are medications that may be used to treat hypertension. Match each medication with the correct classification.

Medication

_____ Hydrochlorothiazide (HydroDIURIL)

_____ Furosemide (Lasix)

_____ Clonidine (Catapres)

_____ Spironolactone (Aldactone)

_____ Doxazosin (Cardura)

_____ Atenolol (Tenormin)

_____ Carvedilol (Coreg)

_____ Hydralazine (Apresoline)

_____ Benazepril (Lotensin)

_____ Amlodipine (Norvasc)

_____ Valsartan (Diovan)

Classification

a. Beta-adrenergic blockers

b. Angiotensin-converting enzyme inhibitors

c. Thiazide diuretics

d. Angiotensin II receptor blocker

e. Loop diuretics

f. Aldosterone receptor blockers

g. Alpha-adrenergic blockers

h. Direct vasodilators

i. Calcium channel blockers

j. Mixed alpha- and beta-blockers

k. Central-acting alpha-adrenergic agonists

Exercise 2

Virtual Hospital Activity

45 minutes

- Sign in to work at Pacific View Regional Hospital for Period of Care 1. (*Note:* If you are already in the virtual hospital from a previous exercise, click on **Leave the Floor** and then on **Restart the Program** to get to the sign-in window.)
- From the Patient List, select Patricia Newman (Room 406).
- Click on **Go to Nurses' Station**.
- Click on **Chart** and then on **406**.
- Click on **History and Physical**.
- Click on **Nursing Admission**.

1. Patricia Newman was diagnosed with hypertension 15 years ago. What risk factors for hypertension does she have?

2. Chlorothiazide has been prescribed to manage Patricia Newman's hypertension. Review the Virtual Hospital Drug Guide. Which characteristics and descriptions are correct in regard to this medication? Select all that apply.

   _____ Monitor for orthostatic hypotension

   _____ Administer before bed

   _____ May cause vertigo, headache, and weakness

   _____ Associated with an increase in libido

   _____ May cause metabolic acidosis

   _____ Assess patient's weight, intake, and output daily

   _____ Thiazide diuretic

3. Patricia Newman has been prescribed atenolol. A nurse recognizes that the medication should be held if

   the systolic blood pressure is less than _____ or the heart rate is less than _____.

4. When planning care, a nurse must recognize that which of the following imbalances may occur as a result of administering chlorothiazide?
   a. Hypoglycemia
   b. Hypokalemia
   c. Hypocalcemia
   d. Hypouricemia

5. _____ When caring for a patient who has been prescribed chlorothiazide, the nurse recognizes that the patient is at an increased risk for digoxin toxicity. (True/False)

- Click on **Return to Nurses' Station**.
- Click **EPR** and then on **Login**.
- Select **406** from the Patient drop-down menu and **Vital Signs** from the Category drop-down menu. Use the arrows at the bottom of the screen to view previously recorded data.

6. What are Patricia Newman's documented blood pressure measurements since admission?

7. Is her prescribed antihypertensive medication effectively treating her hypertension at this point?

8. Based on her most recent blood pressure readings, in which of the following blood pressure classifications would you place Patricia Newman?
   a. Normal systolic
   b. Prehypertension
   c. Hypertension, stage 1
   d. Hypertension, stage 2

- Click on **Return to Nurses' Station**.
- Click on **406** at the bottom of the screen.
- Click on **Patient Care** and then on **Nurse-Client Interactions**.
- Select and view the video titled **0740: Evaluation—Response to Care**. (*Note:* Check the virtual clock to see whether enough time has elapsed. You can use the fast-forward feature to advance the time by 2-minute intervals if the video is not yet available. Then click again on **Patient Care** and **Nurse-Client Interactions** to refresh the screen.)

9. What might be contributing to Patricia Newman's elevated blood pressure at this point?

- Click on **Chart** and then on **406**.
- Click on **History and Physical**.
- Review the physician documentation for the Review of Systems.

10. What indicates that this patient is in need of further teaching regarding hypertension?

- Click on **Patient Education**.

11. What additional educational goals related to the management of her hypertension would be appropriate for Patricia Newman?

12. Patricia Newman indicates that she does not participate in any exercise programs. Which of the following recommendations concerning exercise have been identified to reduce hypertension?
    a. Participate in high-intensity aerobic physical activity for at least 45 minutes each day for at least 3 days per week.
    b. Participate in moderate-intensity aerobic activity for at least 20 minutes a day for at least 2 days per week.
    c. Participate in 30 minutes of moderate-intensity exercise most days of the week, with a goal of 150 minutes per week.
    d. Participate in low-intensity exercise lasting at least 30 minutes 6 times per week.

13. Patricia Newman indicates that she does not exercise because she feels fatigued. When discussing sodium restrictions with her, which of the following recommendations best reflects the amount of sodium that she should have in her daily diet intake?
    a. Less than or equal to 1200 mg
    b. Less than or equal to 1500 mg
    c. Less than or equal to 2300 mg
    d. Less than or equal to 2500

14. In addition to maintaining a good exercise routine and diet, patients should be advised to limit the

    amount of alcohol consumed. Individuals should drink no more than _____ oz of beer,

    _____ oz of wine, and _____ oz of 80-proof whiskey per day.

Exercise 3

Virtual Hospital Activity

40 minutes

- Sign in to work at Pacific View Regional Hospital for Period of Care 1. (*Note:* If you are already in the virtual hospital from a previous exercise, click on **Leave the Floor** and then on **Restart the Program** to get to the sign-in window.)
- From the Patient List, select Harry George (Room 401).
- Click on **Go to Nurses' Station**.
- Click on **EPR** and then on **Login**.
- Select **401** from the Patient drop-down menu and **Vital Signs** from the Category drop-down menu. Use the arrows at the bottom of the screen to view previously recorded data.

1. Document Harry George's blood pressure results below.

	Tues 0305	Tues 0705	Tues 1105	Tues 1505	Tues 1905	Tues 2305	Wed 0305	Wed 0705
Blood pressure								

- Click on **Exit EPR**.
- Click on **Chart** and then on **401**.
- Click on **History and Physical**.

2. Does Harry George have a history of hypertension?

3. Does he have any risk factors for hypertension? If yes, please identify.

4. Based on the blood pressure results recorded in question 1, in which classification of hypertension would you put Harry George's blood pressure?

5. For what potential complications should you assess Harry George related to untreated hypertension?

- Click on **Diagnostic Reports** and review the reports.
- Click on **Laboratory Reports** and review the results.

6. Several diagnostic tests were ordered by the physician to help identify target organ disease. In column 2 of the table below, identify the target organ disease that the test screens for and the specific findings that would indicate damage caused by hypertension. In column 3, record Harry George's results. Finally, in column 4, indicate whether these results provided evidence of the target organ disease identified in column 2.

Diagnostic Test	Target Organ Disease and Findings Suggestive of Damage Caused by Hypertension	Harry George's Results	Any Evidence of Target Organ Disease?
Chest x-ray			
BUN			
Creatinine			
Urinalysis			

7. Listed below are several classifications of medication that could be used to manage Harry George's elevated blood pressures. Match each drug classification with its corresponding mechanism of action.

Drug Classification	Mechanism of Action
_____ Thiazide and related diuretics	a. Inhibit Na^+-retaining and K^+-excreting effects of aldosterone in the distal and collecting tubules
_____ Loop diuretics	b. Inhibit NaCl reabsorption in the ascending limb of the loop of Henle; increase excretion of Na^+ and Cl^-
_____ Potassium-sparing diuretics	c. Reduce systemic vascular resistance and blood pressure by direct arterial vasodilation
_____ Aldosterone receptor blockers	
_____ Central-acting alpha-adrenergic antagonists	d. Block movement of calcium into cells, resulting in vasodilation
_____ Angiotensin-converting enzyme inhibitors	e. Inhibit NaCl reabsorption in the distal convoluted tubule; increase excretion of Na^+ and Cl^-; decrease ECF volume
_____ Calcium channel blockers	f. Inhibit conversion of angiotensin I to angiotensin II
_____ Direct vasodilators	g. Reduce K^+ and Na^+ exchange in the distal and collecting tubules; result in decreased excretion of potassium and sodium
_____ Angiotensin II receptor blockers	h. Reduce sympathetic outflow; reduce peripheral sympathetic tone, producing vasodilation and decreasing SVR and BP
	i. Block action of angiotensin II and produce vasodilation and increased Na^+ and water excretion

8. What symptoms might Harry George display if his systolic blood pressure dramatically increased above 180 mm Hg or his diastolic blood pressure increased above 110 mm Hg?

9. What determines the seriousness of the patient's condition in hypertensive emergency?

10. What measurement will the health care team use to guide and evaluate therapy during a hypertensive emergency? Describe the initial goal of therapy.

11. Describe the interprofessional and nursing management of a patient with a hypertensive emergency.

Atrial Fibrillation

Reading Assignment: Dysrhythmias (Chapter 35)

Patient: Piya Jordan, Room 403

Goal: To utilize the nursing process to competently care for patients with dysrhythmias.

Objectives:

1. Describe telemetry rhythm strip characteristics of atrial fibrillation.
2. Identify potential etiologic causes of atrial fibrillation for an assigned patient.
3. Assess a patient for clinical manifestations of atrial fibrillation.
4. Develop a plan of care to monitor a patient for potential complications of atrial fibrillation.
5. Perform appropriate assessments before administering pharmacologic therapy for atrial fibrillation.
6. Accurately administer IV digoxin.
7. Discuss the use of anticoagulation therapy for a patient with atrial fibrillation.
8. Develop appropriate educational outcomes for a patient with a history of atrial fibrillation.

In this lesson, you will learn the essentials of caring for a patient with a cardiac dysrhythmia. You will explore the patient's history, evaluate presenting symptoms and treatment, provide appropriate nursing interventions, and plan an appropriate patient educational outcome related to the dysrhythmia. Piya Jordan is a 68-year-old female admitted with nausea, vomiting, and abdominal pain.

Exercise 1

Writing Activity

20 minutes

1. Describe the conduction pathway of a normal cardiac impulse.

2. Below, match each cardiac event with its corresponding wave or measured interval.

Cardiac Event	**Wave/Interval**
_____ Atrial depolarization	a. P wave
_____ The time required for complete ventricular depolarization and repolarization	b. T wave
	c. QRS wave
_____ The period of time when the impulses spread through the atria, AV node, bundle of His, and Purkinje fibers	d. PR interval
	e. QT interval
_____ Ventricular repolarization	
_____ Ventricular depolarization	

3. Define the following terms.

   a. Automaticity

   b. Contractility

   c. Conductivity

   d. Excitability

   e. Absolute refractory phase

4. List the ten steps recommended by your textbook for a systematic approach to assessing cardiac rhythms.

   (1)

   (2)

   (3)

   (4)

   (5)

   (6)

   (7)

   (8)

   (9)

   (10)

5. What three questions should be considered when evaluating a patient's cardiac rhythms?

   (1)

   (2)

   (3)

Exercise 2

Virtual Hospital Activity

35 minutes

- Sign in to work at Pacific View Regional Hospital for Period of Care 1. (*Note:* If you are already in the virtual hospital from a previous exercise, click on **Leave the Floor** and then on **Restart the Program** to get to the sign-in window.)
- From the Patient List, select Piya Jordan (Room 403).
- Click on **Go to Nurses' Station**.
- Click on **403** at the bottom of the screen.

1. What information regarding cardiovascular status is obtained on initial observation of this patient?

2. Telemetry monitoring is the observation of a patient's heart _____ and

_____ at a site distant from the patient to rapidly identify

_____, _____, or _____.

3. What is atrial fibrillation?

4. Describe the rhythm strip you would expect to see on Piya Jordan's monitor.

5. How does normal sinus rhythm (NSR) differ from atrial fibrillation?

6. Describe the clinical significance of atrial fibrillation in terms of the physiologic consequences of this rhythm.

- Click on **Patient Care** and then on **Physical Assessment**. Complete a focused assessment by clicking on the body system categories (yellow buttons) and body system subcategories (green buttons).

7. Does Piya Jordan exhibit any symptoms of decreased cardiac output related to the atrial fibrillation? If so, describe the symptoms. If not, how would you explain that?

8. If Piya Jordan's heart rate increases, how might the atrial fibrillation affect her blood pressure? Include the physiologic rationale for your answer.

9. For what specific complication related to atrial fibrillation is Piya Jordan at increased risk?

Exercise 3

Virtual Hospital Activity

45 minutes

- Sign in to work at Pacific View Regional Hospital for Period of Care 1. (*Note:* If you are already in the virtual hospital from a previous exercise, click on **Leave the Floor** and then on **Restart the Program** to get to the sign-in window.)
- From the Patient List, select Piya Jordan (Room 403).
- Click on **Go to Nurses' Station**.
- Click on **MAR** and then click on tab **403**.

1. What medication is prescribed to treat Piya Jordan's atrial fibrillation? Review the Drug Guide and describe the therapeutic effects of this medication as related to atrial fibrillation.

2. Why did the physician order a digoxin level when the patient first presented to the Emergency Department with a chief complaint of abdominal pain, nausea, and vomiting? (*Hint:* Review her presenting symptoms, as well as the Drug Guide.)

- Click on **Return to Room 403**.
- Click on **Chart** and then on **403**.
- Click on **Laboratory Reports**.

3. Review Piya Jordan's digoxin level on Monday at 2200. The reported level can best be considered:
   a. low.
   b. therapeutic.
   c. toxic.

4. When performing an assessment of Piya Jordan, the nurse must be cognizant of the signs of digoxin toxicity. Review the VCE Drug Guide. Which of the following manifestations are consistent with digoxin toxicity? Select all that apply.

   _____ Tachycardia

   _____ Hypertension

   _____ Elevated temperature

   _____ Bradycardia

   _____ Seeing halos of light around bright objects

   _____ Photophobia

   _____ Anorexia

   _____ Weakness

   _____ Drowsiness

   _____ Depression

   _____ Nausea

   _____ Diarrhea

5. Piya Jordan's potassium level on admission to the Emergency Department on Monday at 2200 was

   _____ mEq/L.

6. How does this relate to possible digoxin toxicity?

- Click on **History and Physical**.

7. What other medication was prescribed for Piya Jordan related to atrial fibrillation before this admission? Explain the rationale for this medication.

- Click on **Physician's Orders**.

8. On Tuesday at 0130 the physician ordered which medication preoperatively to reverse Piya Jordan's anticoagulation? Identify the medication ordered on Tuesday at 0800 to reverse her anticoagulation. How would you know whether this was effective? Please explain.

9. What was ordered postoperatively to prevent clot formation?

- Click on **Nursing Admission**.
- Scroll down to the Health Promotion section.

10. What knowledge (or lack of) does Piya Jordan verbalize regarding her history of atrial fibrillation?

- Click on **Patient Education** and review the goals for Piya Jordan.

11. What might you add to these goals based on your answer to question 10?

12. How would treatment for Piya Jordan differ if her atrial fibrillation had been a new acute onset and the physician was trying to return her to a normal sinus rhythm rather than just control her heart rate?

13. What diagnostic procedure would you expect to be performed before cardioversion? Why?

14. Several treatment options that may be used for patients with recurrent or sustained atrial fibrillation that is not responsive to medical management. Below, match each treatment option with its description.

Treatment Option	**Description**
_____ AV nodal ablation	a. A procedure that is done in an EPS laboratory and involves placing a catheter in the right atrium; a low-voltage, high-frequency form of electrical energy ablates (destroys) the ectopic foci.
_____ Maze procedure	b. Destruction of the AV node and insertion of a permanent ventricular pacemaker.
_____ Radiofrequency catheter ablation	c. Surgical procedure where incisions are made in both atria and cryotherapy (cold therapy) is used to stop the formation and conduction of ectopic foci.

- Click on **Return to Nurses' Station**.
- Click on **Medication Room**.
- Click on **MAR** to determine medications that Piya Jordan is ordered to receive at 0800. (*Note:* You may click on **Review MAR** at any time to verify correct medication order. Remember to look at the patient's name on the MAR to make sure you have the correct record. You must click on the correct room number within the MAR. Click on **Return to Medication Room** after reviewing the correct MAR.)
- Based on your care for Piya Jordan, access the various storage areas of the Medication Room to obtain the necessary medications you need to administer.
- For each area you access, first select the medication you plan to administer, then click on **Put Medication on Tray**. When finished with a storage area, click on **Close Drawer**.
- Click on **View Medication Room**.
- Click on **Preparation** and choose the correct medication to administer.
- Click on **Prepare** and then on **Next**.
- Choose the correct patient to administer this medication to. Click on **Finish**.
- Repeat the above three steps until all medications that you want to administer are prepared.
- You can click on **Review Your Medications** and then on **Return to Medication Room** when you are ready. Once you are back in the Medication Room, you can go directly to Piya Jordan's room by clicking on **403** at the bottom of the screen.
- Administer the medication(s) utilizing the six rights of medication administration. After you have collected the appropriate assessment data and are ready for administration, click on **Patient Care** and then on **Medication Administration**. Verify that the correct patient and medication(s) appear in the left-hand window. Then click the down arrow next to Select. From the drop-down menu, select **Administer** and complete the Administration Wizard by providing any information requested.
- When the Wizard stops asking for information, click on **Administer to Patient**.
- Specify **Yes** when asked whether this administration should be recorded in the MAR.
- Finally, click on **Finish**.

15. Over how many minutes would you administer the IV digoxin?

16. What should you have assessed before administering digoxin to Piya Jordan today?

Now let's see how you did!

- Click on **Leave the Floor** at the bottom of your screen.
- From the Floor Menu, select **Look at Your Preceptor's Evaluation**.
- Click on **Medication Scorecard**.

17. Note below whether or not you correctly administered the appropriate medication(s). If not, why do you think you were incorrect? According to Table C in this scorecard, what resources should be used and what important assessments should be completed before administering the medication(s)? Did you utilize these resources and perform these assessments correctly?

Venous Thromboembolism (Deep Vein Thrombosis and Pulmonary Embolism)

Reading Assignment: Lower Respiratory Problems (Chapter 27)
Vascular Disorders (Chapter 37)

Patient: Clarence Hughes, Room 404

Goal: To utilize the nursing process to competently care for patients with venous thromboembolism (VTE).

Objectives:

1. Describe factors that increase the risk of developing a venous thromboembolism (VTE).
2. Identify nursing interventions to reduce the risk of VTE in hospitalized patients.
3. Identify clinical manifestations of pulmonary embolism.
4. Prioritize nursing care for a patient with acute onset of respiratory distress and chest pain.
5. Describe diagnostic testing relative to the diagnosis of pulmonary embolism.
6. Describe pharmacologic therapy for a patient with pulmonary embolism.
7. Accurately calculate the correct dosage of heparin for a patient using a sliding scale.

In this lesson, you will learn the essentials of caring for a patient diagnosed with an acute pulmonary embolism that resulted from a venous thromboembolism (VTE). You will explore the patient's history, evaluate presenting symptoms and treatment, provide appropriate nursing interventions, and assess the patient's progress throughout the clinical day. Clarence Hughes is a 73-year-old male admitted for an elective left knee arthroplasty.

Exercise 1

Writing Activity

15 minutes

1. Explain the difference between superficial vein thrombosis and venous thromboembolism (VTE).

2. What is Virchow's triad? Identify predisposing conditions for each of the three factors.

3. Describe nursing interventions used to prevent VTE in at-risk patients.

Exercise 2

Virtual Hospital Activity

30 minutes

- Sign in to work at Pacific View Regional Hospital for Period of Care 2. (*Note:* If you are already in the virtual hospital from a previous exercise, click on **Leave the Floor** and then on **Restart the Program** to get to the sign-in window.)
- From the Patient List, select Clarence Hughes (Room 404).
- Click on **Get Report** and review the reports.
- Click on **Go to Nurses' Station**.
- Click on **404** at the bottom of the screen.

1. What is your initial observation as you enter his room?

2. What should your priority actions be at this point?

- Click on **Patient Care** and then on **Nurse-Client Interactions**.
- Select and view the video titled **1115: Interventions—Airway**. (*Note:* Check the virtual clock to see whether enough time has elapsed. You can use the fast-forward feature to advance the time by 2-minute intervals if the video is not yet available. Then click again on **Patient Care** and **Nurse-Client Interactions** to refresh the screen.)

3. Describe the nursing actions in the video. Was it acceptable that the nurse left the patient to go get oxygen? Why or why not? If not, what else could she have done?

4. When assessing Clarence Hughes' lung sounds, what sound is consistent with a pulmonary embolism? Select all that apply.

_____ Clear

_____ Diminished

_____ Crackles

_____ Wheezes

_____ Rhonchi

5. What manifestations are consistent with a pulmonary embolism? Select all that apply.

_____ Sudden onset of dyspnea

_____ Feeling of impending doom

_____ Bradycardia

_____ Hemoptysis

_____ Bradypnea

_____ Change in mental status

- Click on **Chart** and then on **404**.
- Click on **History and Physical**.

6. Based on the patient's history and reason for hospitalization, what risk factors for VTE does he have?

- Click on **Physician's Orders**.

7. Look at the orders for Wednesday at 1120. Document these orders and provide a rationale for each.

Physician's Order	Rationale

- Click on **Return to Room 404**.
- Click on **Patient Care** and then on **Nurse-Client Interactions**.
- Select and view the video titled **1135: Change in Patient Condition**. (*Note:* Check the virtual clock to see whether enough time has elapsed. You can use the fast-forward feature to advance the time by 2-minute intervals if the video is not yet available. Then click again on **Patient Care** and **Nurse-Client Interactions** to refresh the screen.)

8. As the nurse is explaining care to the family, she states that a transporter will be coming to take the patient for a ventilation-perfusion scan. Would you send him down to radiology with only the transporter? Why or why not?

Exercise 3

Virtual Hospital Activity

30 minutes

- Sign in to work at Pacific View Regional Hospital for Period of Care 3. (*Note:* If you are already in the virtual hospital from a previous exercise, click on **Leave the Floor** and then on **Restart the Program** to get to the sign-in window.)
- From the Patient List, select Clarence Hughes (Room 404).
- Click on **Go to Nurses' Station**.
- Click on **Chart** and then on **404**.
- Click on and review the **Laboratory Reports** and **Diagnostic Reports** sections of the chart.

1. Below and on the next page, document the results of the lab tests (from Wednesday 1130) and diagnostic imaging studies ordered for Clarence Hughes.

Diagnostic Test	Result
D-dimer	
PT	
INR	
PTT	

Diagnostic Test	Result
CBC	
Arterial blood gas	
Chest x-ray	
Spiral CT	
Ventilation-perfusion scan	
Venous Doppler study	

2. Based on the above results, what would you conclude to be the cause of Clarence Hughes' acute respiratory distress?

3. What other diagnostic testing could the physician have ordered related to Clarence Hughes' pulmonary embolism? Explain the usefulness and/or significance of each test.

- Click on **Physician's Orders**.

4. What orders were written on Wednesday at 1250 to treat Clarence Hughes' pulmonary embolism?

5. What lab test will be used to titrate the heparin infusion? What are the normal values for this test?

6. What is the desired therapeutic level for this test?

- Click on **Return to Nurses' Station**.
- Click on **MAR** and select tab **404**.

7. Calculate the units of heparin required to administer for the bolus dose.

8. Calculate the infusion rate you would set the IV pump to infuse this medication.

- Click on **Return to Nurses' Station**.
- Click on **Chart** and then on **404**.
- Click on **Laboratory Reports**.

9. What were the results of the PTT and INR at 1300 today? Why were these tests ordered before starting the heparin?

- Click on **Return to Nurses' Station**.
- Click on **404** to enter Clarence Hughes' room.
- Click on **Patient Care** and then on **Nurse-Client Interactions**.
- Select and view the video titled **1510: Disease Management**. (*Note:* Check the virtual clock to see whether enough time has elapsed. You can use the fast-forward feature to advance the time by 2-minute intervals if the video is not yet available. Then click again on **Patient Care** and **Nurse-Client Interactions** to refresh the screen.)

10. When Clarence Hughes' son asks the nurse whether the pulmonary embolism will delay his father's discharge, the nurse states that the heparin takes 2 days to stabilize. Does this mean that the patient will be discharged on heparin? If not, what medication will be used to minimize clot formation? Explain why the patient is not started on this medication rather than heparin.

11. Which lab test will be used to monitor the therapeutic effect of warfarin? What is the therapeutic range for this test?

12. For what possible complications related to the pulmonary embolism would you monitor Clarence Hughes?

Exercise 4

Virtual Hospital Activity

30 minutes

- Sign in to work at Pacific View Regional Hospital for Period of Care 4. (*Note:* If you are already in the virtual hospital from a previous exercise, click on **Leave the Floor** and then on **Restart the Program** to get to the sign-in window.)
- Click on **Chart** and then on **404**. (*Remember:* You are not able to visit patients or administer medications during Period of Care 4. You are able to review patients' records only.)
- Click on **Laboratory Reports**.

1. What is the PTT result for 1900?

- Click on **Physician's Orders**.

2. Based on this result, what would you do now with the heparin infusion? Calculate the infusion rate and the bolus dose needed, if any.

- Click on **Return to Nurses' Station**.
- Click on **Kardex** and then on tab **404**. Review the stated outcomes for Clarence Hughes.

3. Should other outcomes be added because of his pulmonary embolism? Give rationale.

4. What is the expected mortality rate within the first hour of a pulmonary embolism?

5. Describe nursing interventions for patients taking anticoagulants that should be implemented while the patient is receiving heparin therapy.

6. What surgical treatment would be needed if Clarence Hughes' condition were to deteriorate? Explain.

7. If the patient develops another pulmonary embolism, what further treatment might the physician consider to prevent the recurrence of pulmonary emboli? Explain.

17 —————————————————————————

Nutritional Problems

————————————————————————————

Reading Assignment: Nutritional Problems (Chapter 39)

Obesity (Chapter 40)

Patients: Harry George, Room 401

Jacquline Catanazaro, Room 402

Piya Jordan, Room 403

Goal: To utilize the nursing process to competently care for patients with nutritional disorders.

Objectives:

1. Identify patients at risk for malnutrition.
2. Perform a nutritional screening assessment on assigned patients.
3. Evaluate laboratory findings in relation to a patient's nutritional status.
4. Plan appropriate dietary interventions for a patient with malnutrition.
5. Identify a patient's risk factors related to obesity.
6. Formulate an appropriate patient education plan for an overweight patient.

In this lesson, you will learn the essentials of caring for patients with nutritional disorders. You will explore each patient's history, perform a nutritional screening assessment, evaluate findings, and plan appropriate nursing interventions, including the patient's educational needs. Harry George is a 54-year-old male with a 4-year history of type 2 diabetes admitted with infection and swelling of his left foot. Piya Jordan is a 68-year-old female admitted with nausea and vomiting for several days following weeks of poor appetite and increasing weakness. Jacquline Catanazaro is a 45-year-old female admitted with an acute exacerbation of asthma.

Exercise 1

Writing Activity

10 minutes

1. The average person should consume _____ to _____ calories per kilogram of body weight each day to maintain body weight.

2. The nurse is planning an educational program concerning nutrition. Which of the following facts may be included? Select all that apply.

_____ At least half of the daily intake should be from protein sources.

_____ Fat intake should be limited to 20% to 35% of the daily caloric intake.

_____ Fats provide a major source of energy for the body.

_____ Grains, potatoes, and legumes are good sources of complex carbohydrates.

_____ Proteins are needed for growth and repair of body tissues.

3. Describe the difference between complete and incomplete proteins. Give examples of each.

4. Identify and describe the three types of factors that influence obesity.

Exercise 2

Virtual Hospital Activity

40 minutes

- Sign in to work at Pacific View Regional Hospital for Period of Care 1. (*Note:* If you are already in the virtual hospital from a previous exercise, click on **Leave the Floor** and then on **Restart the Program** to get to the sign-in window.)
- From the Patient List, select Harry George (Room 401) and Piya Jordan (Room 403).
- Click on **Go to Nurses' Station**.
- Click on **Chart** and then on **401** for Harry George's chart.
- Click on **History and Physical**.

1. What risk factors for malnutrition are noted in Harry George's History and Physical?

- Click on **Return to Nurses' Station**.
- Click on **Chart** and then on **403** for Piya Jordan's chart.
- Click on **History and Physical**.

2. What risk factors for malnutrition are noted in Piya Jordan's History and Physical?

- Click on **Return to Nurses' Station**.
- Click on **401** at the bottom of the screen.
- Click on **Patient Care**.

3. Although not every patient needs a complete nutritional assessment, it is essential to assess at-risk patients for symptoms of malnutrition. Referring to Table 39-7 in your textbook, assess Harry George for any of the identified findings associated with malnutrition. Obtain subjective information by reading his History and Physical, Nursing Admission form, and laboratory results. Gather the objective data by completing a physical assessment on the patient. Document your findings in column 2 below and on the next two pages. (*Note:* You will perform a similar assessment on Piya Jordan during Exercise 3 and record those findings in column 3.)

Screening Assessments	Harry George	Piya Jordan
Subjective Data Past health history		
Medications		
Surgery or other treatments		

Screening Assessments	Harry George	Piya Jordan

Functional Health Patterns

Health-Perception

Nutritional-Metabolic

Elimination

Activity-Exercise

Cognitive-Perceptual

Role-Relationship

Sexual-Reproductive

Objective Data

General

Integumentary

Eyes

Screening Assessments	Harry George	Piya Jordan
Respiratory		
Cardiovascular		
Gastrointestinal		
Neurologic		
Musculoskeletal		
Laboratory findings		

4. Calculate Harry George's body mass index (BMI) based on his current height and weight by using the following formula:

$$\frac{\text{Weight in pounds}}{\text{Height in inches x Height in inches}} \times 703 = \text{BMI}$$

5. Evaluate the results of your findings in questions 3 and 4. What clinical manifestations of protein-calorie malnutrition does Harry George display?

6. Is Harry George's protein-calorie malnutrition (PCM) primary or secondary? Explain how you came to your conclusion.

Exercise 3

Virtual Hospital Activity

40 minutes

- Sign in to work at Pacific View Regional Hospital for Period of Care 1. (*Note:* If you are already in the virtual hospital from a previous exercise, click on **Leave the Floor** and then on **Restart the Program** to get to the sign-in window.)
- From the Patient List, select Harry George (Room 401) and Piya Jordan (Room 403).
- Click on **Go to Nurses' Station**.
- Click on **403** to enter Piya Jordan's room.
- Click on **Patient Care**.

1. Now perform the same nutritional screening assessment on Piya Jordan as you did for Harry George in the previous exercise. Referring to Table 39-7 in your textbook, assess the patient for any of the identified findings associated with malnutrition. Obtain subjective information by reading her History and Physical, Nursing Admission form, and Laboratory Reports. Acquire the objective data by completing a physical assessment. Document your findings in column 3 of the table in question 3 of Exercise 2.

2. Calculate Piya Jordan's BMI based on her current height and weight by using the following formula:

$$\frac{\text{Weight in pounds}}{\text{Height in inches x Height in inches}} \times 703 = \text{BMI}$$

3. Evaluate the results of your findings for questions 1 and 2. What clinical manifestations of protein-calorie malnutrition, if any, does Piya Jordan display?

4. Is Piya Jordan's protein-calorie malnutrition (PCM) primary or secondary? Explain how you came to your conclusion.

5. Compare and contrast your findings for Harry George and Piya Jordan. What are the similarities? What are the differences?

6. What other laboratory tests, not ordered for either of these patients, might be useful in evaluating their nutritional status?

7. Identify two nursing diagnoses related to Piya Jordan's and Harry George's malnourished status.

8. What type of diet or dietary supplements would you recommend for these two patients?

9. What additional nursing interventions would be appropriate to address these patients' nutritional needs?

Exercise 4

Virtual Hospital Activity

30 minutes

- Sign in to work at Pacific View Regional Hospital for Period of Care 2. (*Note:* If you are already in the virtual hospital from a previous exercise, click on **Leave the Floor** and then on **Restart the Program** to get to the sign-in window.)
- From the Patient List, select Jacquline Catanazaro (Room 402).
- Click on **Go to Nurses' Station**.
- Click on **Chart** and then on **402**.
- Click on **Nursing Admission**.

1. Document Jacquline Catanazaro's current height and weight below.

2. Calculate her BMI using the following formula:

$$\frac{\text{Weight in pounds}}{\text{Height in inches x Height in inches}} \times 703 = \text{BMI}$$

3. Is Jacquline Catanazaro's nutritional status underweight, normal, overweight, obese, or morbidly obese?

- Click on **History and Physical**.

4. What complication of obesity does this patient suffer from?

5. Identify other complications Jacquline Catanazaro may be at risk for related to the categories listed below and on the next page.

Cardiovascular

Respiratory

Metabolic

Musculoskeletal

Liver/gallbladder

Gastrointestinal

Genitourinary

Reproductive

Psychologic

Cancer

6. What measurement could be used to assess Jacquline Catanazaro's risk for cardiovascular complications? Explain the significance of this measurement.

7. What are the contributing factors for Jacquline Catanazaro's increased weight?

- Click on **Return to Nurses' Station**.
- Click on **MAR** and then on tab **402**.

8. Do any of the medications ordered for Jacquline Catanazaro cause weight gain? If so, describe. Consult the Drug Guide provided in the Nurses' Station.

- Click on **Return to Nurses' Station**.
- Click on **402** at the bottom of the screen.
- Click on **Patient Care** and then on **Nurse-Client Interactions**.
- Select and view the video titled **1140: Compliance—Medications**. (*Note:* Check the virtual clock to see whether enough time has elapsed. You can use the fast-forward feature to advance the time by 2-minute intervals if the video is not yet available. Then click again on **Patient Care** and **Nurse-Client Interactions** to refresh the screen.)

9. What concern does the patient voice regarding her medications?

10. Evaluate the nurse's response. Was it appropriate? Accurate?

11. What else could the nurse have suggested to help the patient lose weight?

12. What medications might be used as adjuncts to a diet and exercise program for Jacquline Catanazaro?

13. Is Jacquline Catanazaro a candidate for bariatric surgery? Why or why not?

14. If this patient were morbidly obese, what other treatment options might she have?

Intestinal Obstruction/ Colorectal Cancer

Reading Assignment: Lower Gastrointestinal Problems (Chapter 42)

Patient: Piya Jordan, Room 403

Goal: To utilize the nursing process to competently care for patients with lower gastrointestinal problems.

Objectives:

1. Correlate a patient's history and clinical manifestations with a diagnosis of intestinal obstruction.
2. Evaluate laboratory and diagnostic test results of a patient admitted with a noninflammatory intestinal disorder.
3. Plan appropriate nursing interventions for a patient with a nasogastric tube.
4. Prioritize nursing care for a patient with an intestinal obstruction.
5. Provide appropriate psychosocial interventions for a patient and family diagnosed with colon cancer.
6. Formulate an appropriate patient education plan for a postoperative patient with colorectal cancer.

In this lesson, you will learn the essentials of caring for a patient admitted with an intestinal obstruction and diagnosed with colorectal cancer. You will explore the patient's history, evaluate presenting symptoms and treatment, plan appropriate nursing interventions, and develop an individualized teaching plan. Piya Jordan is a 68-year-old female admitted with nausea and vomiting for several days following weeks of poor appetite and increasing weakness.

Exercise 1

Writing Activity

15 minutes

1. Describe the pathophysiology of fluid and electrolyte imbalances associated with an intestinal obstruction.

2. Compare and contrast mechanical and nonmechanical intestinal obstructions.

   a. Mechanical obstruction

   b. Nonmechanical obstruction

3. The patient suspected of having a bowel obstruction experiences sudden onset of severe, constant abdominal pain. Upon palpation, the abdomen is rigid. Identify potential causes of these manifestations. Select all that apply.

   _____   The bowel has perforated.

   _____   The patient has peritonitis.

   _____   The bowel is strangulated.

   _____   The bowel is telescoping.

   _____   The patient has a gastrointestinal virus.

4. How does the removal of polyps help to prevent colorectal cancer?

5. Identify the four most common sites of metastasis for colorectal cancer.

_____ Brain

_____ Liver

_____ Kidneys

_____ Bones

_____ Lungs

_____ Peritoneum

_____ Regional lymph nodes

Exercise 2

Virtual Hospital Activity

40 minutes

- Sign in to work at Pacific View Regional Hospital for Period of Care 1. (*Note:* If you are already in the virtual hospital from a previous exercise, click on **Leave the Floor** and then on **Restart the Program** to get to the sign-in window.)
- From the Patient List, select Piya Jordan (Room 403).
- Click on **Go to Nurses' Station**.
- Click on **Chart** and then on **403**.
- Click on **Emergency Department** and review the ED physician's Progress Note.
- Click on **History and Physical** and review the record.

1. What were Piya Jordan's presenting symptoms? What history of symptoms is recorded?

- Click on **Laboratory Reports**.

2. Document Piya Jordan's admission chemistry results below. Evaluate whether each of the results is normal, decreased, or increased. Offer your rationale for any abnormalities in the last column.

	Monday 2200	Decreased, Normal, or Increased?	Rationales for Abnormality
Sodium			
Potassium			
Creatinine			
BUN			
Albumin			
Protein			
Alkaline phosphatase			

- Click on **Diagnostic Reports**.

3. What was the result of the patient's KUB?

4. Piya Jordan has a small bowel obstruction. When considering the typical manifestations of a small bowel obstruction, which of the following is most characteristic?
   a. Frequent and copious vomiting
   b. Gradual onset
   c. Absolute constipation
   d. Abdominal distention is slight

5. Why do you think a CT scan of the abdomen was ordered? What was the result?

6. What part of the bowel is the terminal ileum?

7. Was Piya Jordan's obstruction mechanical or nonmechanical? Explain.

8. For which priority problem related to intestinal obstruction should a nurse assess Piya Jordan?
   a. Renal complications
   b. Fluid and electrolyte deficiencies
   c. Anemia
   d. Increased risk for pulmonary embolus

9. If the patient had sought medical attention before the obstruction worsening, what other diagnostic testing might she have undergone? Explain what the test would show.

- Click on **History and Physical**.
- Click on **Emergency Department** and review the ED physician's Progress Note.
- Click on **Laboratory Reports** and review admission test results.

10. Now that you know Piya Jordan has a colonic mass, let's look at her presenting symptoms again. Common clinical manifestations of colorectal cancer are listed below. Place an X next to each sign or symptom consistent with the patient's history and her physical examination findings on admission.

_____ Rectal bleeding

_____ Alternating constipation and diarrhea

_____ Anemia

_____ Blood in stools

_____ Weakness

_____ Colicky abdominal pain

_____ Vague abdominal discomfort

_____ Sensation of incomplete emptying

_____ Ribbon-like stools

_____ Weight loss

- Click on **Physician's Orders**.

11. What IV fluid did the Emergency Department physician initially order on Monday at 2115? Why? Considering Piya Jordan's initial vital signs in the Emergency Department record, provide the rationale for the IV fluid order.

12. What else did the Emergency Department physician order on Tuesday at 0015 to treat the intestinal obstruction? Explain the purpose of this intervention.

- Click on **Return to Nurses' Station**.
- Click on **403** at the bottom of the screen.
- Click on **Patient Care** and then on **Physical Assessment**. Complete a focused assessment by clicking on the body system categories (yellow buttons) and the body system subcategories (green buttons).

13. Document the findings from your focused gastrointestinal assessment below.

14. Describe any additional assessments and/or interventions related to the nasogastric tube that you might do for Piya Jordan.

Exercise 3

Virtual Hospital Activity

45 minutes

- Sign in to work at Pacific View Regional Hospital for Period of Care 3. (*Note:* If you are already in the virtual hospital from a previous exercise, click on **Leave the Floor** and then on **Restart the Program** to get to the sign-in window.)
- From the Patient List, select Piya Jordan (Room 403).
- Click on **Go to Nurses' Station**.
- Click on **Chart** and then on **403**.
- Click on **History and Physical**.

1. Below is a list of risk factors for colorectal cancer. Place an X next to those that are documented in Piya Jordan's record. Select all that apply.

_____ Age over 50 years

_____ Familial adenomatosis polyposis (FAP)

_____ Alcohol intake (4 or more drinks a week)

_____ Red meat intake (7 or more servings a week)

_____ Inflammatory bowel disease

_____ Family history of colorectal cancer (first degree relative)

_____ Cigarette smoking

_____ Hereditary nonpolyposis colorectal cancer syndrome (HNPCC)

_____ Obesity (body mass index greater than 30 kg/m^2)

_____ Male gender

_____ Diabetes mellitus

_____ Colorectal polyps

- Click on **Laboratory Reports**.

2. Below, document Piya Jordan's hemoglobin and hematocrit on admission. How would you explain the results?

	Monday 2200	Decreased, Within Normal Limits, or Increased?	Rationale for Abnormality
Hemoglobin			
Hematocrit			

- Click on **Expired MARs**.

3. What was ordered on Tuesday at 0130 and administered preoperatively to clean out Piya Jordan's bowel?

- Click on **Surgical Reports**.

4. Review the Report of Operation. Name and describe the surgical procedure.

5. What is the most likely cell type for Piya Jordan's cancer?

6. How will the physician know what kind of cancer the tumor is?

7. Based on the surgeon's description in the operative report, explain how you would classify Piya Jordan's tumor according to the following two staging systems.

   a. Dukes Classification System

   b. TNM Classification

- Click on **Laboratory Results**.

8. Why did the physician order an amylase, lipase, and liver function tests? What do the results demonstrate?

- Click on **Return to Nurses' Station** and then on **403** at the bottom of the screen.
- Click on **Patient Care** and then on **Nurse-Client Interactions**.
- Select and view the video titled **1500: Preventing Complications**. (*Note:* Check the virtual clock to see whether enough time has elapsed. You can use the fast-forward feature to advance the time by 2-minute intervals if the video is not yet available. Then click again on **Patient Care** and **Nurse-Client Interactions** to refresh the screen.)

9. What nursing interventions are discussed during this brief video? Why are they appropriate for Piya Jordan?

- Click on **Patient Care** and then on **Nurse-Client Interactions**.
- Select and view the video titled **1540: Discharge Planning**. (*Note:* Check the virtual clock to see whether enough time has elapsed. You can use the fast-forward feature to advance the time by 2-minute intervals if the video is not yet available. Then click again on **Patient Care** and **Nurse-Client Interactions** to refresh the screen.)

10. Piya Jordan's daughter seems to be overwhelmed by her mother's illness and needs. Describe psychosocial interventions that the nurse might plan to help Piya Jordan and her daughter.

11. What would you teach Piya Jordan's daughter regarding health promotion and prevention of colon cancer for herself? Select all that apply.

_____ Increasing physical activity and having a diet rich in fruits, vegetables, and grains may decrease the risk for colorectal cancer.

_____ A fecal occult blood test (FOBT) or fecal immunochemical test (FRT) is indicated every 5 years.

_____ A diet rich in red meat has been shown to decrease colorectal cancer risk.

_____ Long-term NSAID use may reduce the risk for colorectal cancer.

_____ Colonoscopy is recommended every 10 years, beginning at age 40.

LESSON 19

Diabetes Mellitus, Part 1

Reading Assignment: Diabetes Mellitus (Chapter 48)

Patient: Harry George, Room 401

Goal: To utilize the nursing process to competently care for patients with diabetes mellitus.

Objectives:

1. Describe the etiology of type 1 and type 2 diabetes mellitus.
2. Compare and contrast the characteristics of type 1 and type 2 diabetes.
3. Identify the relationship between diabetes and other disease processes.
4. Evaluate a patient's risk factors for diabetes.
5. Assess a patient for short- and long-term complications of diabetes.
6. Develop an appropriate plan of care for a patient with type 2 diabetes.

In this lesson, you will learn the essentials of caring for a patient admitted with complications related to diabetes mellitus. You will explore the patient's history, evaluate presenting symptoms and treatment, plan appropriate nursing interventions, and develop an individualized teaching plan. Harry George is a 54-year-old male with a 4-year history of type 2 diabetes, admitted with infection and swelling of his left foot.

Exercise 1

Writing Activity

5 minutes

1. Below, identify each of the characteristics as indicative of type 1 or type 2 diabetes mellitus.

Characteristic	**Type of Diabetes**
_____ Pancreas produces some insulin	a. Type 1 diabetes mellitus
_____ Gradual onset	b. Type 2 diabetes mellitus
_____ Autoimmune	
_____ Associated with obesity	
_____ The most common type of diabetes	
_____ Characterized by ketosis at onset of disease	
_____ More common in young people	
_____ Insulin resistance	
_____ Often asymptomatic	
_____ Islet cell autoantibodies	

Exercise 2

Virtual Hospital Activity

45 minutes

- Sign in to work at Pacific View Regional Hospital for Period of Care 1. (*Note:* If you are already in the virtual hospital from a previous exercise, click on **Leave the Floor** and then on **Restart the Program** to get to the sign-in window.)
- From the Patient List, select Harry George (Room 401).
- Click on **Go to Nurses' Station**.
- Click on **Chart** and then on **401**.
- Click on **History and Physical**.

1. What risk factors for diabetes are noted in Harry George's family history?

2. Describe the history of this patient's present illness.

3. What is the relationship between the infection in Harry George's foot and his diabetes mellitus?

- Click on **Laboratory Reports**.

4. Upon admission Harry George's blood glucose level was _____ mg/dL.

5. What abnormalities in his urinalysis results can be attributed to the diabetes? Explain the relationship.

- Click on **Emergency Department**.
- Scroll down to read the Emergency Department physician's notes for 1345.

6. What factor in Harry George's recent history most likely contributed to his hyperglycemia?

- Click on **Nursing Admission**.

7. Listed below are clinical manifestations of diabetes mellitus that are identified in the textbook. In column 2, indicate (with Yes or No) whether each manifestation is usually present in type 2 diabetes. In column 3, indicate (with Yes or No) whether Harry George displays each manifestation based on the nurse's initial assessment.

Clinical Manifestations	Present in Type 2 DM? (Yes or No)	Experienced by Harry George? (Yes or No)
Polyuria		
Polydipsia		
Polyphagia		
Visual changes		
Weakness/fatigue		
Weight loss		
Chronic complications		
Recurrent infections		
Prolonged wound healing		

8. To what extent does Harry George fit the typical picture of a patient with type 2 diabetes mellitus?

- Click on **Return to Nurses' Station** and then on **401** at the bottom of the screen.
- Click on **Patient Care** and then on **Nurse-Client Interactions**.
- Select and view the video titled **0755: Disease Management**. (*Note:* Check the virtual clock to see whether enough time has elapsed. You can use the fast-forward feature to advance the time by 2-minute intervals if the video is not yet available. Then click again on **Patient Care** and **Nurse-Client Interactions** to refresh the screen.)

9. What does Harry George tell the nurse about his appetite?

10. What diet has been ordered for the patient?

11. When planning the diet for Harry George, which of the following recommendations should be implemented?
    a. The largest component of the daily intake should consist of proteins.
    b. Trans and saturated fat intake should be minimized.
    c. Consume no more than one serving of fish per week.
    d. Fiber intake of a patient with diabetes should be less than that of a nondiabetic.

12. Indicate whether each of the following statements is true or false.

    a. _____ Alcohol intake is strictly prohibited for the patient with diabetes.

    b. _____ Alcohol intake can result in sharp episodes of hyperglycemia for patients who are on oral hypoglycemics or insulin therapies.

Exercise 3

Virtual Hospital Activity

40 minutes

- Sign in to work at Pacific View Regional Hospital for Period of Care 2. (*Note:* If you are already in the virtual hospital from a previous exercise, click on **Leave the Floor** and then on **Restart the Program** to get to the sign-in window.)
- From the Patient List, select Harry George (Room 401).
- Click on **Go to Nurses' Station**.
- Click on **Chart** and then on **401**.
- Click on **Laboratory Reports**.
- Click on **Physician's Orders**.

1. The physician has ordered an HbgA1c. This test is best used to:
   a. assess overall glucose control over the past 2 to 3 months.
   b. assess compliance with insulin or oral hypoglycemic therapies for the past 30 days.
   c. assess the presence of early vascular complications.
   d. assess for insulin resistance in older adults.

2. What is the normal range for an HbgA1c test?
   a. 0% to 1.5%
   b. 2% to 4%
   c. 4% to 6%
   d. 7% to 9%

3. What factors can affect the accuracy of the fasting plasma glucose (FPG) test? Select all that apply.

   _____ Ingestion of narcotic pain medications

   _____ Patient age

   _____ Failure of the patient to fast before the test

   _____ Activity restrictions

   _____ Corticosteroid use

   _____ Bed rest

4. Review Harry George's HbgA1C results. What are his results? What does this indicate about his condition?

5. What implication does the patient's issue of poor glycemic control have for his future?

- Click on **Return to Nurses' Station** and then on **401** at the bottom of the screen.
- Click on **Patient Care** and then on **Physical Assessment**. Complete a head-to-toe assessment by clicking on the body system categories (yellow buttons) and body system subcategories (green buttons).

6. Below, document any abnormal results from your assessment of Harry George.

Assessment Area	Assessment Results
Head & Neck	
Chest	
Back & Spine	
Upper Extremities	
Abdomen	
Pelvic	
Lower Extremities	

- Click on **EPR** and then on **Login**.
- Select **401** from the Patient drop-down menu and **Neurologic** from the Category drop-down menu. Use the arrows at the bottom of the screen to view previously recorded data.

7. List any abnormal results from the neurologic and cardiovascular assessment on Monday at 1835.

8. Describe the potential long-term complications of diabetes mellitus below.

Macrovascular

Diabetic retinopathy

Neuropathy

Nephropathy

9. Harry George is beginning to exhibit signs of which of the following complications of diabetes mellitus? Select all that apply.

_____ Neuropathy

_____ Nephropathy

_____ Retinopathy

_____ Microvascular disorders

_____ Peripheral vascular disease

10. What patient teaching would you plan to offer this patient to prevent further injury secondary to reduced sensation in his left foot?

11. Using correct NANDA format, state three nursing diagnoses related to Harry George's diabetes.

Diabetes Mellitus, Part 2

Reading Assignment: Diabetes Mellitus (Chapter 48)

Patient: Harry George, Room 401

Goal: To utilize the nursing process to competently administer medications prescribed to treat patients with diabetes mellitus.

Objectives:

1. Describe the pharmacologic therapy used for a patient with diabetes.
2. Evaluate a patient's response to insulin therapy.
3. Assess a patient for side effects of insulin therapy.
4. Describe the clinical manifestations of hypoglycemia as a side effect of insulin therapy.
5. Develop an individualized teaching plan for a patient with type 2 diabetes.

In this lesson, you will learn the essentials regarding pharmacologic therapy for a patient admitted with complications related to diabetes mellitus. You will identify, describe, administer, and evaluate effects of prescribed antidiabetic medications. Harry George is a 54-year-old male with a 4-year history of type 2 diabetes, admitted with infection and swelling of his left foot.

Exercise 1

Writing Activity

30 minutes

1. Identify and describe the various types of insulin by completing the table below.

Insulin Classification/ Generic Name	Brand Name	Onset (hour)	Peak (hour)	Duration (hour)
Rapid-acting: aspart				
lispro				
glulisine				

Insulin Classification/ Generic Name	Brand Name	Onset (hour)	Peak (hour)	Duration (hour)
Short-acting: regular insulin				
Intermediate-acting: NPH				
Long-acting: glargine				
determir				
degludac				
Inhaled insulin				

2. Match each classification of oral hypoglycemic agents with its corresponding mechanism of action.

Classification

_____ Alpha-glucosidase inhibitors

_____ Biguanides

_____ Dipeptidyl peptidase-4 inhibitors

_____ Dopamine receptor agonists

_____ Meglitinides

_____ Sodium glucose cotransporter 2 inhibitors

_____ Sulfonylureas

_____ Thiazolidinediones

Mechanism of Action

a. First-line treatment for type 2 diabetes. Reduce glucose production by liver; enhance glucose uptake by tissues, especially muscles.

b. Insulin sensitizers. Improve insulin sensitivity, transport, and utilization at target tissues; do not increase insulin production.

c. Primary action is to increase insulin production. Also decrease glucose production and enhance cellular sensitivity to insulin.

d. Rapidly absorbed and eliminated. Increase insulin production during and after the meal, mimicking normal blood glucose response to eating.

e. Starch blockers taken with the first bite of each meal. Slow absorption of carbohydrates in small intestine; lower postprandial glucose levels.

f. Decrease renal glucose reabsorption and increase urinary excretion of glucose.

g. Enhance activity of incretins to stimulate insulin production and decrease hepatic glucose production.

h. Activate dopamine receptors and lower glucose levels by an unknown mechanism.

3. Identify and describe two non-insulin injectable pharmacologic agents useful in treating diabetes mellitus.

Exercise 2

Virtual Hospital Activity

40 minutes

- Sign in to work at Pacific View Regional Hospital for Period of Care 1. (*Note:* If you are already in the virtual hospital from a previous exercise, click on **Leave the Floor** and then on **Restart the Program** to get to the sign-in window.)
- From the Patient List, select Harry George (Room 401).
- Click on **Go to Nurses' Station**.
- Click on **Chart** and then on **401**.
- Click on **Physician's Orders**.

1. What medication was ordered to control Harry George's diabetes on Monday at 1345?

2. At what point after administering Harry George's regular insulin will he be at the greatest risk for hypoglycemia?
   a. 30 minutes to 1 hour after administration
   b. 2 to 5 hours after administration
   c. 4 to 12 hours after administration
   d. 12 to 18 hours after administration

3. What was the sliding scale insulin order? Provide both the glucose levels and insulin doses.

- Click on **Return to Nurses' Station**.
- Click on **Kardex** and then on **401** for Harry George's record.

4. According to the Kardex, how often should the capillary blood glucose be tested?

- Click on **Return to Nurses' Station**.
- Click on **MAR** and then on tab **401**.

5. According to the MAR, when should the insulin sliding scale be administered? What was the time of this order?

6. What would you do regarding the inconsistencies identified above?

7. What problems might you anticipate for Harry George if he does not receive insulin coverage at bedtime?

- Click on **Return to Nurses' Station** and then on **401** at the bottom of the screen.
- Click on **Clinical Alerts**.

8. Harry George's fasting morning glucose is 206 mg/dL. This manifestation may be explained by which of the following? Select all that apply.

_____ The dusk to dawn effect

_____ The Somogyi effect

_____ The dawn phenomena

_____ The insulin rebound effect

_____ The side effects of antibiotics

Prepare and administer the sliding scale insulin for this glucose level by following these steps:

- Click on **Medication Room** on the bottom of the screen.
- Click on **MAR** or on **Review MAR** at any time to verify how much insulin to administer based on sliding scale. (*Hint:* Remember to look at the patient's name on the MAR to make sure you have the correct records and to click on the correct room number within the MAR.) Click on **Return to Medication Room** after reviewing the correct MAR.
- Click on **Unit Dosage** and then on drawer **401** for Harry George's medications.
- Select **Insulin Regular**, click on **Put Medication on Tray**, and then click on **Close Drawer**.
- Click on **View Medication Room**.
- Click on **Preparation** and choose the correct medication to administer. Click on **Prepare**.
- Click on **Next**, choose the correct patient to administer this medication to, and click on **Finish**.
- You can click on **Review Your Medications** and then on **Return to Medication Room** when ready. Once you are back in the Medication Room, you can go directly to Harry George's room by clicking on **401** at the bottom of the screen.
- Click on **Patient Care**.
- Click on **Medication Administration** and follow the steps in the Administration Wizard to complete the insulin administration.

9. How much insulin should be administered?

10. What is the preferred site of administration for fastest absorption?

11. Fill in the chart below regarding the insulin you just administered.

	Expected Length of Time	Actual Time after 0730 Dose
Onset		
Peak		
Duration		

12. When performing the assessments on Harry George, which of the following manifestations, if present, may be indicative of hypoglycemia? Select all that apply.

_____ Diaphoresis

_____ Irritability

_____ Bradycardia

_____ Hunger

_____ Hypertension

_____ Visual disturbances

_____ Weakness

13. While you are preparing to administer Harry George's insulin, he asks you why he is taking this because he did not use insulin at home. How would you answer him?

14. For what side effects related to the current insulin regimen should you monitor Harry George?

Exercise 3

Virtual Hospital Activity

40 minutes

- Sign in to work at Pacific View Regional Hospital for Period of Care 4. (*Note:* If you are already in the virtual hospital from a previous exercise, click on **Leave the Floor** and then on **Restart the Program** to get to the sign-in window.)
- Click on **Chart** and then on **401**. (*Remember:* You are not able to visit patients or administer medications during Period of Care 4. You are able to review patients' records only.)
- Click on **Nurse's Notes**.

1. Glyburide has been prescribed for Harry George. To which of the following classifications does this medication belong?
   a. Alpha-glucosidases
   b. Meglitinides
   c. Sulfonylureas
   d. Biguanides

2. Read the notes for Wednesday at 1730. What does Harry George request regarding glyburide?

3. How would you respond to the patient's demands?

4. How often was he supposed to take the glyburide at home?

5. How often is the glyburide to be administered during his admission?

6. Why do you think the frequency was increased in the hospital? What concerns might you have regarding this increase? (*Hint:* Patient is also receiving insulin.)

7. According to your textbook, which two main glyburide side effects should you assess Harry George for?

8. Why is Harry George not a candidate for treatment with metformin?

9. What patient teaching related to diabetes would be appropriate for Harry George?

- Click on **Go to Nurses' Station**.
- Click on **Chart** and then on **401**.
- Click on **Nurse's Notes**.

10. Below, chart Harry George's blood glucose level and insulin administration since admission to the medical-surgical unit. (*Hint:* Scroll to the bottom of the Nurse's Notes and begin with Monday at 2030.)

Date/Time	Blood Glucose Level	Amount of Regular Insulin Administered
Monday 2030		
Tuesday 0730		
Tuesday 1130		
Tuesday 1800		
Tuesday 2300		
Wednesday 0730		
Wednesday 1130		
Wednesday 1730		

11. Based on Harry George's pattern of blood glucose levels, would you evaluate his current therapy as effective? If not, how might the physician further treat the patient's diabetes?

12. What concern with Harry George's care in question 10 is the nurse ethically and legally bound to report?

LESSON **21** ———————————————————

Osteomyelitis

Reading Assignment: Musculoskeletal Problems (Chapter 63)

Patient: Harry George, Room 401

Goal: To utilize the nursing process to competently care for patients with osteomyelitis.

Objectives:

1. Describe the pathophysiology of osteomyelitis.
2. Assess an assigned patient for clinical manifestations of osteomyelitis.
3. Describe the causative agent and category of osteomyelitis in an assigned patient.
4. Safely administer IV antibiotic therapy as prescribed for osteomyelitis.
5. Evaluate diagnostic tests related to osteomyelitis.
6. Develop an individualized discharge plan of care for a patient with osteomyelitis complicated by other disease processes and homelessness.

In this lesson, you will learn the essentials of caring for a patient diagnosed with osteomyelitis. You will explore the patient's history, evaluate presenting symptoms and treatment, administer prescribed medications, and develop an individualized discharge teaching plan. Harry George is a 54-year-old male admitted with infection and swelling of his left foot, a history of type 2 diabetes, alcohol abuse, and nicotine addiction.

Exercise 1

Writing Activity

10 minutes

1. Describe the pathophysiology of osteomyelitis.

243

2. The most common causative organism of osteomyelitis is _____.

Exercise 2

Virtual Hospital Activity

45 minutes

- Sign in to work at Pacific View Regional Hospital for Period of Care 2. (*Note:* If you are already in the virtual hospital from a previous exercise, click on **Leave the Floor** and then on **Restart the Program** to get to the sign-in window.)
- From the Patient List, select Harry George (Room 401).
- Click on **Go to Nurses' Station**.
- Click on **Chart** and then on **401**.
- Click on **History and Physical**.

1. The clinical manifestations of osteomyelitis can include both local and systemic symptoms, the most common of which are listed below. Which of these signs or symptoms are consistent with Harry George's history and his physical examination findings on admission? Select all that apply.

    _____   Constant bone pain

    _____   Swelling

    _____   Tenderness

    _____   Warmth at infection site

    _____   Restricted movement

    _____   Fever

    _____   Night sweats

    _____   Chills

    _____   Restlessness

    _____   Nausea

    _____   Malaise

2. Which of the factors in Harry George's medical/personal history may have contributed to the development of osteomyelitis? Select all that apply.

    _____   Type 2 diabetes mellitus

    _____   Homelessness

    _____   Alcoholism

    _____   History of orthopedic surgery

    _____   Advancing age

3. Describe how Harry George's chronic osteomyelitis could have developed from a direct entry source and an indirect entry source. Provide rationale for each source of entry.

- Click on **Physician's Orders**.

4. The following tests are useful in the diagnosis and evaluation of osteomyelitis. Match each test with its corresponding description.

Diagnostic Test	**Description**
_____ MRI and CT scan	a. Initial test to determine causative organism
_____ Wound culture	b. Positive in the area of infection
_____ White blood cell count	c. Most definitive way to determine causative organism
_____ X-ray of affected extremity	d. Elevated results of this test indicate infection
_____ Radionuclide bone scan	e. Used to help identify the extent of the infection, including soft tissue involvement
_____ Bone/tissue biopsy	f. Changes with this test do not appear early in the course of the disease
_____ Erythrocyte sedimentation rate (ESR)	g. Elevated with inflammatory process

5. Place an X next to each diagnostic test that was performed on admission for Harry George. Select all that apply.

_____ MRI and CT scan

_____ Wound culture

_____ White blood cell count

_____ X-ray of affected extremity

_____ Radionuclide bone scan

_____ Bone/tissue biopsy

_____ Erythrocyte sedimentation rate (ESR)

- Click on **Diagnostic Reports**.

6. Compare the reports with the pathophysiology of osteomyelitis as described in your textbook. What findings documented on these reports are consistent with osteomyelitis? What do these findings mean?

Findings documented on the x-ray report

Findings documented on the bone scan

Meaning of both

- Click on **Return to Nurses' Station**.
- Click on **MAR** and then on tab **401**.

7. Determine what routine medications (excluding the continuous IV and insulin coverage) you will be giving to Harry George during the day shift (0700-1500). Below, list his medication orders in the left column. For each order, identify the drug classification, the reason why the drug is given, and the time it is due. You may refer to the Drug Guide by returning to the Nurses' Station and clicking on the **Drug** icon in the lower left corner of your screen.

Medication Order	Classification	Reason for Giving	Time Due

8. Which medication was Harry George receiving that was discontinued on Tuesday?

- Click on **Return to Nurses' Station**.
- Click on **Chart** and then on **401**.
- Click on **Physician's Orders**.

9. What new medication replaced the discontinued medication that you identified in question 9?

- Click on **Physician's Notes**.

10. Why was this change in medication ordered?

- Click on **Laboratory Reports**.

11. You are aware that antibiotics have been ordered for Harry George because of his leg infection. You decide to check the white blood cell results because you are curious (also, you are sure your nursing instructor will ask you about it). Document the white blood cell results for the times specified below and indicate whether each result is normal, elevated, or decreased. Then indicate the trend of the lab results in the last column.

Tests	Monday 1500	Normal, Elevated, Decreased?	Tuesday 1100	Normal, Elevated Decreased?	Overall Trend — Stable, Increasing, or Decreasing?
Total white blood cell count					
Neutrophil segs					
Neutrophil bands					
Lymphocytes					
Monocytes					
Eosinophils					
Basophils					

12. Explain the meaning of the white blood cell results in the table above, including the overall direction of the change in the white blood cell count and the significance of this change.

- Click on **Return to Nurses' Station**.
- Click on **Patient List**.
- Click on **Get Report** for Harry George. Review the report.

13. Is there anything else you wish the nurse would have included in the report regarding osteomyelitis? If so, what?

- Click on **Return to Nurses' Station**.
- Click on **Medication Room**.
- Click on **IV Storage**.
- Click on the **Small Volume** bin and choose the IV antibiotic that is due to be given at 0800.

14. What dilution of this IV antibiotic is available for you to administer?

15. Over what amount of time should you infuse the IV antibiotic? You may refer to the Drug Guide for this information.

16. If you are using an IV pump to deliver this medication piggyback, what rate (mL per hour) will you select to give this infusion?

Exercise 3

Virtual Hospital Activity

40 minutes

- Sign in to work at Pacific View Regional Hospital for Period of Care 2. (*Note:* If you are already in the virtual hospital from a previous exercise, click on **Leave the Floor** and then on **Restart the Program** to get to the sign-in window.)
- From the Patient List, select Harry George (Room 401).
- Click on **Go to Nurses' Station** and then on **401** at the bottom of the screen.
- Inside the patient's room, click on **Take Vital Signs**.

1. Record the vital sign findings below.

BP	SpO$_2$	Temp	HR	RR	Pain

- Click on **Patient Care** and then on **Physical Assessment**.
- Click on **Lower Extremities** and complete a focused neurovascular assessment related to osteomyelitis by clicking on the body system categories (yellow buttons) and body system subcategories (green buttons).

2. Below, record the results of your assessment.

- Click on **Patient Care** and then on **Nurse-Client Interactions**.
- Select and view the video titled **1120: Wound Management**. (*Note:* Check the virtual clock to see whether enough time has elapsed. You can use the fast-forward feature to advance the time by 2-minute intervals if the video is not yet available. Then click again on **Patient Care** and **Nurse-Client Interactions** to refresh the screen.)

3. How does the nurse describe the progress of Harry George's wound condition? How does the patient respond?

4. Based on your findings from questions 1 through 3, identify three priority nursing diagnoses for Harry George.

- Click on **Kardex** and then on tab **401**.

5. What interventions noted on the Kardex are related to Harry George's osteomyelitis?

- Click on **Return to Room 401**.
- Click on **Medication Room**.
- Click on **MAR** to determine what medications you need to administer to Harry George during this time period (1115-1200).
- Click on **Return to Medication Room**.
- Click on **IV Storage**.
- Click on the **Small Volume** bin and choose the IV antibiotic that is due to be given at 1200.
- Click on **Put Medication on Tray**.
- Click on **Close Bin**.
- Click on **View Medication Room**.
- Click on the **Drug** icon in the lower left corner of the screen.

6. Look up gentamicin in the Drug Guide and read the alert under Administration and Handling. What must you assess before administering this drug?

- Click on **Return to Medication Room**.
- Click on **Nurses' Station**.
- Click on **Chart** and then on **401**.
- Click on **Laboratory Reports**.

7. Harry George's most recent gentamicin peak level is _____ mcg/L, and his most recent gentamicin

   trough level is _____ mcg/L.

8. Based on these results, what should your nursing actions be?

9. According to the Drug Guide, what toxic side effects of gentamicin must you monitor for? List the assessments needed to monitor for each side effect.

Ototoxicity

Nephrotoxicity

Neurotoxicity

10. What types of follow-up diagnostic tests should be anticipated for Harry George to determine how well the osteomyelitis is responding to therapy? What changes will occur in these diagnostic test results if therapy is effective?

11. If Harry George's infection does not respond to the antibiotic therapy, what other interventions will most likely be planned? Explain how these would benefit him.

12. The treatment of chronic osteomyelitis may continue for up to _____.

13. Based on what you know and have read, what do you expect will be included in Harry George's discharge instructions and follow-up care to manage his osteomyelitis?

14. Based on this patient's current living conditions, how do you think his care might best be managed?

Chronic Low Back Pain

Reading Assignment: Musculoskeletal Problems (Chapter 63)

Patient: Jacquline Catanazaro, Room 402

Goal: To utilize the nursing process to competently care for patients with an intervertebral disk problem.

Objectives:

1. Describe the pathophysiology of low back pain.
2. Identify clinical manifestations related to low back pain and/or herniated intervertebral disk.
3. Plan appropriate interventions to treat low back pain.
4. Evaluate a patient's potential to comply with a health care management plan.
5. Develop an individualized teaching plan for a patient with low back pain.

In this lesson, you will learn the essentials of caring for a patient experiencing chronic low back pain. You will explore the patient's history, evaluate presenting symptoms and treatment, plan appropriate nursing interventions to treat the patient's symptoms, and develop an individualized discharge teaching plan. Jacquline Catanazaro is a 45-year-old female admitted with an acute exacerbation of asthma.

Exercise 1

Writing Activity

15 minutes

1. List the risk factors for low back pain.

2. Identify five causes of low back pain.

3. Describe the pathophysiology of low back pain caused by degenerative disc disease.

4. Identify the differentiating clinical manifestations below as characteristic of either acute low back pain or chronic low back pain.

Differentiating Clinical Manifestations	**Type**
_____ Lasts 4 weeks or less	a. Acute low back pain
_____ Repeated incapacitating episode	b. Chronic low back pain
_____ Lasts more than 3 months	
_____ Associated with some type of activity that causes undue stress	

5. Below, match each procedure used for the management of back pain with its corresponding description.

Procedure	Description

_____ Intradiscal electrothermoplasty (IDET)

a. A titanium device is surgically placed on the vertebrae, which lifts the vertebrae off a compressed nerve.

_____ Radiofrequency discal nucleoplasty (coblation nucleoplasty)

b. The spine is stabilized by creating an ankylosis (fusion) of adjacent vertebrae with a bone graft from the patient's fibula or iliac crest or from a donated cadaver bone. Bone morphogenetic protein (BMP) may be used instead of bone to stimulate the body to grow new bone at the fusion site.

_____ Interspinous process decompression system (X stop)

c. An outpatient procedure where a needle is inserted into the disc. A radiofrequency probe is used to break up the molecular bonds of the gel in the nucleus pulposus. This causes decompression of the disc, reduction of pressure on nerve roots, and relief of pain.

_____ Laminectomy

_____ Discectomy

d. An artificial disc is inserted through a small incision below the umbilicus after the damaged disc is removed. Restores movement at the level of implant and eliminates pain.

_____ Microsurgical discectomy

_____ Percutaneous discectomy

e. A minimally invasive outpatient procedure involving the insertion of a needle into the affected disc with x-ray guidance. A wire is then threaded through the needle and into the disc. The wire is heated, which denervates the small nerve fibers that have invaded the disc. The heated wire also partially melts the annulus, triggering the body to generate new reinforcing proteins in the fibers of the annulus.

_____ Charite disc implantation

_____ Spinal fusion

f. Surgical removal of part of the posterior arch of the vertebra (known as the lamina) to gain access to and remove the protruding disc.

g. An outpatient procedure using a tube passed through the retroperitoneal soft tissues to the disc with the aid of fluoroscopy. A laser is then used on the damaged portion of the disc.

h. Removal of a herniated disc to decompress the nerve root.

i. A version of standard discectomy utilizing a microscope to allow better visualization of the disc and disc space during surgery to aid in the removal of the damaged portion. Helps maintain bony stability of the spine.

Exercise 2

Virtual Hospital Activity

45 minutes

- Sign in to work at Pacific View Regional Hospital for Period of Care 3. (*Note:* If you are already in the virtual hospital from a previous exercise, click on **Leave the Floor** and then on **Restart the Program** to get to the sign-in window.)
- From the Patient List, select Jacquline Catanazaro (Room 402).
- Click on **Go to Nurses' Station**.
- Click on **Chart** and then on **402**.
- Click on **History and Physical**. Review the section titled History of Present Illness.

1. What are the patient's complaints related to her back?

- Scroll down to the section titled Past Medical History.

2. How does the physician describe this problem?

3. How was this diagnosed?

4. Jacquline Catanazaro's back pain can be classified as which of the following?
   a. Acute
   b. Chronic
   d. Referred
   e. Radicular

5. What treatment has she undergone? Explain the mechanism of action and/or rationale for the treatments.

- Click on **Nursing Admission**.

6. What risk factors does Jacquline Catanazaro have for low back pain and/or degenerative disc disease?

7. What assessments should be completed on this patient in relation to the back pain?

- Click on **Nurse's Notes**.

8. How have the nurses addressed Jacquline Catanazaro's complaint of low back pain?

9. What interventions could you suggest that would be appropriate for this patient's back pain during her hospital stay?

- Click on **History and Physical**.

10. What is the physician's plan regarding this patient's back pain? What type of interventions might be offered by this consult?

11. What formal program described in your textbook might be helpful for Jacquline Catanazaro?

12. What are the two goals for this program?

13. If her pain is not relieved by nonsurgical management, which of the procedures defined in your clinical preparation would you expect to be used for Jacquline Catanazaro? Why?

- Click on **Patient Education**.

14. What goals related to this patient's back pain would you add?

15. When caring for the patient with low back pain, which patient teaching points may be helpful? Select all that apply.

_____ Sleep in a sidelying position with the knees and hips bent, using a pillow between the knees for support

_____ Avoid prolonged standing

_____ Bend at the knees, not the waist, when lifting heavy objects

_____ Sleep on the abdomen with the legs straight

_____ Participate in low-impact aerobic exercise and in strength and flexibility training regularly

_____ Use heat applications as needed

_____ Use cold applications as needed

_____ Place one foot on a low step stool when standing for long periods to avoid back strain

_____ Maintain a healthy body weight

• Click on **History and Physical**.

16. What impact does her schizophrenia have on her back pain?

• Click on **Return to Nurses' Station**.
• Click on **402** at the bottom of the screen.
• Click on **Patient Care** and then on **Nurse-Client Interactions**.
• Select and view the video titled **1540: Discharge Planning**. (*Note:* Check the virtual clock to see whether enough time has elapsed. You can use the fast-forward feature to advance the time by 2-minute intervals if the video is not yet available. Then click again on **Patient Care** and **Nurse-Client Interactions** to refresh the screen.)

17. After viewing the video, what other suggestions do you have for assisting Jacquline Catanazaro with compliance after discharge?

Osteoporosis

Reading Assignment: Musculoskeletal Problems (Chapter 63)

Patient: Patricia Newman, Room 406

Goal: To utilize the nursing process to competently care for patients with osteoporosis.

Objectives:

1. Describe the pathophysiology of osteoporosis.
2. Assess the assigned patient for clinical manifestations of osteoporosis.
3. Describe appropriate pharmacologic therapy for prevention and/or treatment of osteoporosis.
4. Describe the appropriate technique for safe administration of medications used to prevent or treat osteoporosis.
5. Plan appropriate interventions to promote health and prevent further bone loss in a patient with osteoporosis.
6. Develop an individualized teaching plan for an assigned patient with osteoporosis.

In this lesson, you will learn the essentials of caring for a patient diagnosed with osteoporosis. You will explore the patient's history, evaluate presenting symptoms and treatment, administer prescribed medications, and develop an individualized discharge teaching plan. Patricia Newman is a 61-year-old female admitted with pneumonia and a history of emphysema.

Exercise 1

Writing Activity

10 minutes

1. Describe the pathophysiology of osteoporosis.

2. Which of the following are risk factors for the development of osteoporosis? Select all that apply.

_____ Male gender

_____ Over age 30

_____ Family history

_____ Asian ethnicity

_____ Obese

_____ Post menopausal

_____ Sedentary lifestyle

_____ Cigarette smoking

_____ Elevated testosterone

_____ Social use of alcohol

_____ Anticonvulsant medications

Exercise 2

Virtual Hospital Activity

35 minutes

- Sign in to work at Pacific View Regional Hospital for Period of Care 2. (*Note:* If you are already in the virtual hospital from a previous exercise, click on **Leave the Floor** and then on **Restart the Program** to get to the sign-in window.)
- From the Patient List, select Patricia Newman (Room 406).
- Click on **Go to Nurses' Station**.
- Click on **Chart** and then on **406**.
- Click on **History and Physical** and review the record.
- Click on **Nursing Admission** and review this record as well.

1. How long has Patricia Newman been diagnosed with osteoporosis?

2. What modifiable and nonmodifiable risk factors does she have for osteoporosis?

Modifiable risk factors

Nonmodifiable risk factors

3. What diagnostic test would have been ordered to diagnose this patient's osteoporosis? Describe the test and identify results diagnostic for osteoporosis.

4. What clinical manifestation of osteoporosis is documented on the Nursing Admission form?

- Click on **Laboratory Reports**.

5. Do any laboratory results for Patricia Newman correlate with osteoporosis?

6. What other clinical manifestations would you assess Patricia Newman for in relation to osteoporosis?

- Click on **Return to Nurses' Station**.
- Click on **MAR** and then on tab **406**.

7. What medications are ordered for Patricia Newman to help treat and prevent worsening of her osteoporosis? In the table below, identify these medications, their classifications, mechanisms of action, and side effects.

Medication	Drug Classification	Mechanism of Action	Side Effects

Exercise 3

Virtual Hospital Activity

35 minutes

- Sign in to work at Pacific View Regional Hospital for Period of Care 3. (*Note:* If you are already in the virtual hospital from a previous exercise, click on **Leave the Floor** and then on **Restart the Program** to get to the sign-in window.)
- From the Patient List, select Patricia Newman (Room 406).
- Click on **Go to Nurses' Station**.
- Click on **Chart** and then on **406**.
- Click on **Patient Education**.

1. What educational goals already identified could be related to Patricia Newman's osteoporosis?

2. What teaching would you provide for Patricia Newman regarding exercise to prevent further bone loss?

3. Patricia Newman's dietary intake should include a calcium intake of:
   a. 500 mg/day.
   b. 1000 mg/day.
   c. 1200 mg/day.
   d. 1400 mg/day.

4. When planning education for Patricia Newman about the importance of vitamin D and methods to improve calcium absorption, what should be included in the discussion? Select all that apply.

   _____ Calcium is necessary for adequate vitamin D metabolism.

   _____ Exposure to sunlight for 30 to 45 minutes per day is needed to ensure adequate vitamin synthesis.

   _____ The daily recommended vitamin D intake is 800 IU.

   _____ Calcium supplements are best absorbed when taken with meals.

   _____ Calcium carbonate is preferred over calcium gluconate due to a higher amount of elemental calcium.

   _____ Calcium should be taken in large, once-daily doses for the best absorption.

5. Additional treatment options are available for the management of osteoporosis. Listed in the left column below are medications and medication classifications that may be useful in the management of this condition. Match each medication/medication classification with its corresponding method of action.

Classification/Medication	Mechanism of Action
_____ Biphosphonates (Didronel, Fosamax, Aredia, Actonel, Skelid, and Boniva)	a. Inhibits osteoclast-mediated bone resorption, thereby increasing bone mineral density and total bone loss
_____ Selective estrogen receptor modulators (SERMS; e.g., Evista)	b. Increases the action of osteoblasts, stimulating new bone formation
_____ Calcitonin	c. Mimics the effect of estrogen on bone by reducing bone resorption without stimulating the tissues of the breast or uterus
_____ Teriparatide (Forteo)	d. A thyroid hormone that inhibits osteoclastic activity, thus decreasing bone loss

6. In relation to her diagnosis of osteoporosis, Patricia Newman is most at risk for

_____.

- Click on **Return to Nurses' Station** and then on **406** at the bottom of the screen.
- Click on **Patient Care** and then on **Nurse-Client Interactions**.
- Select and view the video titled **1500: Discharge Planning**. (*Note:* Check the virtual clock to see whether enough time has elapsed. You can use the fast-forward feature to advance the time by 2-minute intervals if the video is not yet available. Then click again on **Patient Care** and **Nurse-Client Interactions** to refresh the screen.)

7. Although the discussion in this video was related to the patient's pulmonary disease, how would smoking cessation benefit her musculoskeletal problem?

8. What other health care disciplines might be useful to help Patricia Newman with her discharge needs related to osteoporosis?

9. What psychosocial nursing diagnosis might be a potential problem for this patient related to her slightly stooped posture and going home on oxygen? What nursing interventions would be appropriate to help her with this difficulty?

Osteoarthritis and Total Knee Replacement

Reading Assignment: Musculoskeletal Trauma and Orthopedic Surgery (Chapter 62)
Arthritis and Connective Tissue Diseases (Chapter 64)

Patient: Clarence Hughes, Room 404

Goal: To utilize the nursing process to competently care for patients with osteoarthritis.

Objectives:

1. Describe clinical manifestations and treatment for a patient with debilitating osteoarthritis.
2. Document a focused assessment on a postoperative patient who has undergone a total knee arthroplasty.
3. Plan appropriate interventions to prevent complications related to a total knee replacement in an assigned patient.
4. Identify and provide rationales for collaborative care measures used to treat a patient after a total knee arthroplasty.

In this lesson, you will learn the essentials of caring for a patient undergoing a total knee arthroplasty for treatment of debilitating osteoarthritis. You will document assessments, plan, implement, and evaluate care given. Clarence Hughes is a 73-year-old male admitted for an elective knee replacement. Begin this lesson by reviewing the general concepts of acid-base balance as presented in your textbook.

Exercise 1

Writing Activity

10 minutes

1. Briefly describe the pathophysiology of osteoarthritis (OA).

2. List risk factors related to the occurrence of osteoarthritis.

3. What clinical manifestations are associated with osteoarthritis? Select all that apply.

_____ Fatigue

_____ Fever

_____ Worsening pain with joint use

_____ Localized pain

_____ Stiffness

_____ Unilateral joint involvement

_____ Bouchard's nodes

_____ Heberden's nodes

_____ Systemic organ involvement

_____ Crepitation

4. What laboratory and/or radiographic testing are used in the diagnosis of OA?

Exercise 2

Virtual Hospital Activity

40 minutes

- Sign in to work at Pacific View Regional Hospital for Period of Care 1. (*Note:* If you are already in the virtual hospital from a previous exercise, click on **Leave the Floor** and then on **Restart the Program** to get to the sign-in window.)
- From the Patient List, select Clarence Hughes (Room 404).
- Click on **Go to Nurses' Station**.
- Click on **Chart** and then on **404**.
- Click on **History and Physical**.

1. Which surgical procedure was Clarence Hughes admitted to the hospital for?

2. Describe the symptoms that brought him to this point.

3. According to the History and Physical, what medications and/or treatments have been used to treat Clarence Hughes before he elected to have surgery?

4. According to your textbook, what is the usual indication for total knee arthroplasty?

- Click on **Surgical Reports**.

5. How does the report of operation describe the surgical procedure performed on Clarence Hughes?

6. What medication was added to the cement used for this procedure? Explain the rationale for the use of this medication.

7. What was Clarence Hughes' estimated blood loss (EBL)?

• Click on **Physician's Orders**.
• Scroll down to read the orders for Sunday 1600.

8. What assessments are ordered every 4 hours? Describe specifically how these assessments are completed and what the nurse is looking for.

• Scroll up to read the orders for Monday 0715.

9. What equipment is ordered for Clarence Hughes' left knee? Explain the purpose of this machine.

10. According to your textbook, what could be used to immobilize the operative knee in extension?

- Click on **Return to Nurses' Station**.
- Click on **EPR** and then on **Login**.
- Select **404** from the Patient drop-down menu and **Intake and Output** from the Category drop-down menu.

11. Find "Output: Drain #1" for documentation of Hemovac drainage. How much total drainage is recorded?

12. What were Clarence Hughes' intake and output shift totals on Tuesday at 1500 and 2300? Based on these totals, identify his fluid volume status and provide a rationale for the imbalance.

- Click on **Exit EPR**.
- Click on **Chart** and then on **404**.
- Click on **Laboratory Reports**.

13. What was Clarence Hughes' hemoglobin and hematocrit on Tuesday at 0600?

14. Evaluate Clarence Hughes' admitting hemoglobin and hematocrit, estimated blood loss, Hemovac drainage output, and the 16-hour intake and output on Tuesday. Why do you think his hemoglobin and hematocrit was decreased?

- Click on **Physician's Orders**.

15. What was ordered on Tuesday at 1000 to correct the above laboratory result?

Exercise 3

Virtual Hospital Activity

45 minutes

- Sign in to work at Pacific View Regional Hospital for Period of Care 1. (*Note:* If you are already in the virtual hospital from a previous exercise, click on **Leave the Floor** and then on **Restart the Program** to get to the sign-in window.)
- From the Patient List, select Clarence Hughes (Room 404).
- Click on **Get Report**.

1. What are your concerns for Clarence Hughes after receiving report?

- Click on **Go to Nurses' Station**.
- Click on **404** at the bottom of the screen.
- Click on **Patient Care** and then on **Physical Assessment**. Complete a focused assessment by clicking on the body system categories (yellow buttons) and body system subcategories (green buttons).

2. Document the findings from your focused assessment below.

Area Assessed	Findings

- Click on **Clinical Alerts**.

3. Based on these findings, what would be your priority interventions?

- Click on **Medication Room**.
- Click on **MAR** to determine prn medications that have been ordered for Clarence Hughes to address his constipation and pain. (*Note:* You may click on **Review MAR** at any time to verify the correct medication order. Remember to look at the patient's name on the MAR to make sure you have the correct record. You must click on the correct room number within the MAR. Click on **Return to Medication Room** after reviewing the correct MAR.)
- Click on **Unit Dosage**; from the close-up view, click on drawer **404**.
- Select the medications you would like to administer. After each selection, click on **Put Medication on Tray**. When you are finished selecting medications, click on **Close Drawer**.
- Click on **View Medication Room**.
- Click on **Automated System** (or on the Automated System unit itself). Click on **Login**.
- Select the medication you would like to administer and click on **Put Medication on Tray**. Repeat this process if you wish to administer other medications from the Automated System.
- When you are finished, click on **Close Drawer**. At the bottom right corner of the next screen, click on **View Medication Room**.
- From the Medication Room, click on **Preparation**.
- From the list of medications on your tray, choose the correct medication to administer.
- Click on **Next**.
- Specify the correct patient to administer this medication to and click on **Finish**.
- Repeat the previous three steps until all medications that you want to administer are prepared.
- You can click on **Review Your Medications** and then on **Return to Medication Room** when ready. Once you are back in the Medication Room, you can go directly to Clarence Hughes' room by clicking on **404** at the bottom of the screen.
- Administer the medication utilizing the six rights of medication administration. After you have collected the appropriate assessment data and are ready for administration, click on **Patient Care** and then on **Medication Administration**. Verify that the correct patient and medication(s) appear in the left-hand window. Then click the down arrow next to Select.
- From the drop-down menu, select **Administer** and complete the Administration Wizard by providing any information requested. When the Wizard stops asking for information, click on **Administer to Patient**.
- Specify **Yes** when asked whether this administration should be recorded in the MAR.
- Finally, click on **Finish**. You will evaluate your performance in this area at the end of this exercise (see question 14).

4. What is missing on the patient's order for oxycodone with acetaminophen? What measures need to be taken?

5. Based on the knowledge that most antacids frequently decrease absorption of other medications when concurrently administered, what options might the nurse employ to ensure adequate absorption of pain medication? Consult the Virtual Hospital Drug Guide if needed.

- Click on **Patient Care** and then on **Nurse-Client Interactions**.
- Select and view the video titled **0735: Empathy**. (*Note:* Check the virtual clock to see whether enough time has elapsed. You can use the fast-forward feature to advance the time by 2-minute intervals if the video is not yet available. Then click again on **Patient Care** and **Nurse-Client Interactions** to refresh the screen.)

6. The nurse attempts to appear empathetic by offering to listen to the patient's concerns. Are her actions congruent with her verbal communication? Why or why not?

7. What would you as a student nurse do differently?

8. While planning nursing care for Clarence Hughes, identify five potential complications related to his postoperative status and measures that can be employed to prevent them. Document your plan of care below.

Complications   **Preventative Measures**

- Click on **Chart** and then on **404**.
- Click on **Consultations**.

9. What is the physical therapy team doing for Clarence Hughes?

- Click on **Physician's Orders**.

10. What is the patient's activity order for Wednesday morning?

11. Review the physician's orders from Monday. What is the patient's goal for CPM therapy today (Wednesday)?

12. Review Clarence Hughes' home situation in the nursing admission form. Do you think the ambulation and CPM goals are sufficient for the patient to be discharged tomorrow? Why or why not?

* Click on **Patient Education**.

13. What teaching should be completed for Clarence Hughes before his discharge?

Now let's see how you did during your earlier medication administration!

* Click on **Return to Room 404**.
* Click on **Leave the Floor** at the bottom of your screen.
* From the Floor Menu, click on **Look at Your Preceptor's Evaluation**.
* Click on **Medication Scorecard**.

14. Disregard the report for the routine scheduled medications but note below whether or not you correctly administered the appropriate prn medications. If not, why do you think you were incorrect? According to Table C in this scorecard, what resources should be used, and what important assessments should be completed before administering these medications? Did you utilize these resources and perform these assessments correctly?